MW01222843

Vitamin D:
Antidote to Winter and the Darkness

# Vitamin D:
# Antidote to Winter and the Darkness

Michael D. Merrill, MD, MS

Published 2006 by Lulu.com. ISBN 978-1-4303-0574-3

Printed by Lulu.com in the United States of America

Front Cover: Photo by Hughes L'eglise-Bataille, licensed through Creative Commons. Design by Karen Harkness.

Back Cover: photo by Michael A. Merrill

## Acknowledgments

I thank the late Deneal Amos: "If you are awake in the presence of a master, one moment will show you the way."

For review of the manuscript, thank you to Dr. Paresh Dandona, Bob Ludwig, Maria Scrivani and Meghan Ciesla.

# Table of Contents

Preface: Unnecessary suffering 1
1. Introduction: What's in it for you? 5
 1.1. A note on terminology 6
2. Background on vitamin D 9
 2.1. Human evolution and vitamin D 9
 2.2. Vitamin D in other animals 12
 2.3. History of vitamin D in public health 13
 2.4. It's a steroid hormone 18
 2.5. Vitamin D deficiency currently 20
 2.6. Vitamin D in food 23
 2.7. It's not well studied because of economics 24
 2.8. Approaching vitamin D decisions 26
3. Lack of sunlight is related to chronic illnesses 31
4. Systems and diseases affected by vitamin D 33
 4.1. Brain 33
 4.2. Immune system 35
 4.3. Cancer 38
 4.4. Bone 39
 4.5. Muscle strength 39
 4.6. Pain 41
 4.7. Skin 42
 4.8. Heart 43
 4.9. Obesity 44
 4.10 Height 44
5. Phenomenology: what vitamin D deficiency feels like 47
6. Stories from patients 51
7. Interviews with vitamin D researchers 53
8. Vitamin D is toxic in very high doses 59
9. Getting enough vitamin D 61
10. Ethical considerations 67
11. Vitamin D in human history 69
12. Conclusion 71
Notes 73

# Preface: Unnecessary suffering

I dislike watching people suffer unnecessarily.

It's partly a side effect of medical training, I think. I walk down the street and see more diagnoses than I have the right to see: osteoporosis, depression, sleep apnea, autoimmune disease. The diagnoses become obvious once you know the physical signs well enough, and the gestalt has become part of my thinking. And I know all sorts of tricks that can make people with these diagnoses feel better and live longer, which are things people care about.

But what should I do? Is it my duty to stop every 10th person on the street and talk to them about preventive health? Even if I were to do this only occasionally I would get mixed feedback, including outright hostility. And then people frequently don't believe me. I might be a crackpot, they think, or some kind of nutritional zealot. Even my friends and family sometimes doubt whether I know what I'm talking about, and my message is tossed into the informational soup that they have to sort through every day.

So I'm left with a particular feeling of helplessness and frustration in the midst of the baseline tone of human suffering to which I, by training, am particularly attuned. And I guess I shouldn't complain, but it turns out to be quite painful. So don't laugh at me too hard until you've walked in these shoes.

Of all the many little tricks that can change people's lives, of all the diagnoses that torment people without them knowing it, the one problem that seems to be most pervasive, and causing the most suffering, is vitamin D deficiency.

As an internist, I am a generalist. I deal in how the body's organ systems interact. All through my training, it has struck me that something basic must be wrong with the way we live now. There is just too much malaise, too much achy suffering and depression and absence of health for this to be a normal human state. So for years I have considered everything I have learned from this perspective: can this have something to do with the way things are, this sort of fallen misery in which so many people seem to live?

It is a major public health problem in the United States that no specialty has owned. It cuts across organ systems. And to make it worse, a substance that is not patentable is the remedy – no drug company is going to invest tens of millions in studying it. So there is inadequate data, really, to prove it absolutely to the level to which most physicians are accustomed.

What we inappropriately call "Vitamin D" is actually a steroid hormone within the body – in the same class as cortisone, estrogen and testosterone – that affects every organ system, and most Americans are low in the stuff. It's the anti-hibernation hormone, formed in the skin by sunlight. And we live indoors most of the time now.

Imagine that you were low in your favorite sex hormone. Do you think you'd be feeling any different? Do you think you'd be at your best, that you would be feeling normal? Obviously no. And the pity is that people don't have any sense of what they are missing with vitamin D. They don't know that their mood disturbances, their skin disease, the weird autoimmune disease they have, the "blahs" of modern life in wintertime – all these syndromes might be improved or even cured by vitamin D.

People think I'm crazy when I tell them this. They just smile knowingly and tune me out. Like much of the rest of the information they filter through their heads every day, this message gets tagged "junk" and is forgotten.

Even when I show them a stack of scientific articles, when I tell them the CDC is concerned about the problem, when I tell them that you can get old people out of wheelchairs just by giving them vitamin D, when I tell them that the good feeling they get when they go somewhere sunny on vacation is caused by restoring their vitamin D levels – they still smile, though perhaps a little more uncertainly.

The prophet Ezekiel was warned:

*"When I say unto the wicked, O wicked man, thou shalt surely die; if thou dost not speak to warn the wicked from his way, that wicked man shall die in his iniquity; but his blood will I require at thine hand. Nevertheless, if*

*thou warn the wicked of his way to turn from it; if he does not turn from his way, he shall die in his iniquity; but thou hast delivered thy soul."*

Likewise, please allow me to save myself.

*"Every Morn & every Night*
*Some are Born to sweet Delight.*
*Some are Born to sweet Delight,*
*Some are born to Endless Night."*
- William Blake

# 1. Introduction: What's in it for you?

This book is an argument.

I want to convince you that taking a small dose of vitamin D daily is likely to improve your health. I want to show you that while the evidence for this recommendation is somewhat circumstantial, the body of evidence is large, the risk is minimal and the potential benefits are life-changing and sometimes life-saving.

Traditionally, recommendations like this are the province of the discipline of Public Health – the agencies of the government concerned with preventing and treating widespread disease, like the federal Centers for Disease Control and Prevention. Public Health, however, has bigger problems on its mind at the moment – bioterrorism, emerging global infectious diseases, and epidemics of chronic diseases – and has not focused adequate attention on what many perceive to be merely a superficial nutritional issue.

However, this is not just a nutritional issue. What we call "vitamin D" is a steroid hormone, produced as the sun strikes the skin, affecting every cell of the body. Furthermore, epidemiological studies show that many Americans, especially during the winter and among those living in the North, have deficiencies of this hormone as measured by blood tests. And there is substantial evidence that vitamin D deficiency is a factor in a great many acute and chronic diseases.

What is probably most dramatic, though, is the extent to which supplementing this nutrient can improve one's energy level and sense of well-being, and reduce pain. Vitamin D supplements normalize an endemic problem in the human population living far from the equator: the absence of sunlight. With that problem fixed, whole avenues of energy can open up.

Other potential benefits include:

- Improved overall immune function
- Lower risk of diabetes
- Lower risk of rheumatoid arthritis and lupus, and decreased severity of these diseases if you already have them
- Lower risk of many types of cancer
- Lower risk of osteoporosis, and if you have it, a chance to gain back some bone strength
- Decreased pain
- Increased muscle strength
- Control of skin disease
- Lower blood pressure
- Less chance of schizophrenia in your children
- Children given vitamin D might grow to a taller height

It seems irrational to say that all these benefits might arise from a single substance. Please bear with me, though, and look at the evidence. In the view of some researchers, vitamin D deficiency is probably equivalent to smoking in the magnitude of its effect on one's health.

### 1.1 A note on terminology

The term "vitamin D" actually can refer to a number of separate substances. There is the animal type, naturally occurring in humans, and the plant type, which can be used in humans as a supplement. Each of these types also exists in what I will call an inactive form and an active form. To further complicate matters, there are also vitamin D analogs, chemicals that are similar to the above forms, but tweaked slightly by biochemists in order to create patentable, and therefore marketable, medications.

If the discussion in this section is too dense, please just be aware that when I use the term "vitamin D" in this book, I am referring to the inactive form of vitamin D, either in plant or animal form (as of this writing, the two substances seem relatively interchangeable for practical purposes). Inactive vitamin D is basically the stuff that the body stores up in fatty tissues; it is the strategic vitamin D reserve, so to speak, that is drawn down as necessary.

The animal, inactive form of vitamin D is called cholecalciferol or vitamin D3. Cholecalciferol is created in the skin when ultraviolet light strikes a modified form of cholesterol. After this, the body tacks a hydroxyl group onto the cholecalciferol, making it now 25-hydroxycholecalciferol, and stores it in fatty tissues and in the liver, for later use. Its half life is something like three weeks in the body. Cholecalciferol also is marketed as a nutritional supplement in varying doses up to 2,000 unit tablets or softgels.

The plant-based, inactive form of vitamin D is called ergocalciferol, or vitamin D2. It is a derivative of the plant molecule ergosterol, again made through the action of ultraviolet light. It is processed by the body the same way as cholecalciferol, stored as 25-hydroxyergocalciferol. Ergocalciferol is the type of vitamin D added to milk and many vitamin supplements. Unlike cholecalciferol, ergocalciferol is currently available in a relatively high dose prescription strength of 50,000 unit softgels.

The human body continually needs some vitamin D to function. It is an old hormonal system, hard wired into the most basic elements of our biochemistry. So at a slow, continuous rate, storage-form vitamin D, whether it be manufactured in the skin, or consumed in an animal-based or plant-based supplement, is transformed into active vitamin D. The bulk of this transformation occurs in the kidney, although it occurs in many tissues. This resulting activated vitamin D, called 1,25 – dihydroxycholecalciferol, 1,25-dihydroxyergocalciferol or 1,25-dihydroxy vitamin D, is the most potent steroid hormone in the human body, active at infinitesimal concentrations. These substances cannot be purchased over the counter. There are a few prescription analogs of these, but they are very potent. Taking these substances orally requires careful monitoring, and is usually only necessary for patients with severe kidney disease, who are unable to convert inactive to active vitamin D. Again, when I refer to "vitamin D" in this book, I am referring to vitamin D in its inactive form.

*"It's difficult to get the facts out because there is no sun lobby."*
- Dr. Michael Holick, *The UV Advantage*, 2004.

# 2. Background on Vitamin D

## 2.1. Human evolution and Vitamin D

Human beings evolved in the sun. Modern humans appeared something on the order of 150,000 years ago in Africa, obviously an area with high sun exposure. As such, it is clear that in our evolutionary past, we would have obtained a substantial amount of vitamin D due to regular sun exposure.

Population pressure, the pressure of expanding groups competing for land and resources, pushed humans out of Africa and into Europe and Asia. For those going north, sun exposure diminished. Especially in the winter, weak sunlight at a low angle makes vitamin D synthesis almost impossible.

Humans arriving in the northern areas probably initially had dark skin. Skin color is caused by the pigment melanin, which absorbs and scatters ultraviolet light. The more melanin in the skin, the more difficult it is for ultraviolet light to synthesize the precursor of vitamin D in the skin. As such, the darker skin in the northern latitudes became maladaptive. Or, perhaps more accurately, it became adaptive to develop lighter skin, in order to manufacture vitamin D from sunlight.

In these new arrivals in the north, lower levels of vitamin D meant they would have developed osteoporosis – which has been found in European archaeological sites – along with rickets, immune system dysfunction, seasonal affective disorder, and probably a range of other illnesses. This meant that people with lighter skin in the north were healthier than those with darker skin. Eventually the forces of evolution created what is essentially a partial albinism.

What is fascinating about this is that it occurred over only a few thousand generations. The selective pressure operating on these populations must have been intense for such a rapid change.

A corollary to this idea is that people with darker pigment living at high latitudes today would be at high risk of certain diseases. And in fact we do find high rates of diseases like lupus, multiple sclerosis and several types of cancer in African-American populations living in the north. African-Americans have lower blood vitamin D levels than white people. This is part of the tragedy of the public health problem of vitamin D deficiency: it discriminates racially.

Nina Jablonski and George Chaplin, of the California Academy of Sciences, present a narrative of the evolution of human skin in an article in the Journal of Human Evolution in 2000.[1] Following are points taken from that article.

Scientists have for some time felt that differences in skin pigmentation are likely a reflection of an adaptation to some kind of environmental factor, but have not agreed on what exactly.

Human skin probably started off like that of current chimpanzees, our closest genetic relatives: light or slightly pigmented, with coarse hair covering the entire body. As we evolved the ability to walk on two feet, and as we developed larger brains, we developed the new problem of dissipating great amounts of heat produced by our muscles and brains as they went about their daily metabolism in the heat of Africa. Losing the hair allowed us to dissipate heat more easily, and developing more extensive sweat glands, especially on the face, allowed for increased heat dissipation through evaporative cooling.

But without the hair, the skin was more susceptible to damage from ultraviolet radiation. Damaged skin doesn't dissipate heat well, so the body increased its melanin production to prevent the damage. Melanin causes scattering of incoming radiation, like ultraviolet light, and reduces the amount that reaches the lower levels of the skin, where, for example, the business end of the sweat glands lie. Melanin is also a free radical scavenger, and can decrease the damage done by any ultraviolet light that passes through its area and hits something important.

Now, the only good thing that ultraviolet light does when it hits the skin is produce the vitamin D precursor. Ultraviolet light damages cells and causes mutations. Long term damage to the skin in this manner leads to skin cancers, including basal cell carcinoma, squamous cell carcinoma and melanoma. Ultraviolet light is a carcinogen.

But perhaps the most important effect of ultraviolet light on the skin is its destructive effect on the nutrient folic acid. Folic acid is essential in childbearing-aged women to prevent deformities in developing fetuses. In particular, folic acid prevents spina bifida, a condition in which the spine never closes around the spinal cord, and the nerve tissue is left immediately under the skin, sometimes protruding in a mass outside the curve of the lower back or neck. These children would not have been able to survive in our evolutionary past; these days they can live, but frequently with significant paralysis.

Folic acid is also essential for spermatogenesis, the process in which sperm are created within the male. Drugs affecting folate metabolism have been investigated as male contraceptives, but haven't panned out so far.

Now on the other hand, vitamin D is also essential for human reproduction and well-being. Without adequate vitamin D, severe bony deformities occur in fetuses and children that can be fatal.

So it is clear that there are two forces that would tend to affect, through selective pressure, skin pigmentation in early humans: the ability to protect the body's folic acid stores against degradation by ultraviolet radiation, and the ability to manufacture vitamin D from ultraviolet radiation from sunlight. It turns out that human skin coloration evolves to balance these two forces.

Jablonski and Chaplin gathered information from the literature on skin reflectance, a measure of the absence of skin pigmentation, in indigenous populations around the world. They also collected information on the quantity of ultraviolet light that strikes every point on the earth between 65 degrees north and 65 degrees south latitude, adjusting for factors like elevation and ozone concentrations. It turns out that the more ultraviolet light there is, the darker the skin pigmentation, which is not particularly surprising given that in tropical areas, indigenous people tend to have darker skin.

But it is a subsequent analysis by Jablonski and Chaplin that is most thought-provoking. Based the amount of ultraviolet light needed to make vitamin D, they calculated which areas of the world's surface were bright enough for adequate vitamin D production for various levels of skin pigmentation. They found that for people with light skin, there is insufficient sunlight in Alaska, northern Canada, anywhere north of northern France, and in northern Siberia. For people with dark skin, as in the sub-Saharan African indigenous population, there is insufficient sunlight almost anywhere in the United States, in northern Africa and northwards, and in northern India and northwards.

If these findings are accurate, the implications are profound. For example, they would mean that for dark-skinned African-Americans, it is basically impossible to achieve a healthy level of vitamin D anywhere in the United States without oral supplementation. The findings would also imply that in the most northern areas of Europe, vitamin D deficiency would occur among all peoples without some kind of oral supplementation.

## 2.2 Other animals

The vitamin D pathway in animals appears to have been present for 500 to 700 million years. Everything in the evolutionary tree back to plankton – the tiny little creatures that live in a drop of seawater – produces or consumes vitamin D. Small fish get vitamin D by eating plankton, and then store it; bigger fish get it from smaller fish and store it; marine mammals like walruses get it from fish and store it also. In this way, Vitamin D bioaccumulates – the higher in the food chain, the more of it an animal has. This is analogous to the bioaccumulation in fish of toxins such as mercury. We find low levels of mercury in smaller fish, and sometimes unacceptably high levels in predatory fish like tuna and swordfish. This does not mean that vitamin D is a toxin; on the contrary, this bioaccumulation process may be a more fundamental pathway of which toxins take advantage.

We can see an example of the need for sunlight and vitamin D in iguanas, which are frequently kept as pets. In the wild, these creatures normally spend time sunbathing during the day, partly to regulate body temperature but partly to synthesize vitamin D. Iguanas develop a bone-thinning condition called osteomalacia if they are kept indoors and not exposed to ultraviolet light or fed vitamin D supplements. Vitamin D has become a standard additive to lizard food.

Human populations in the northern latitudes have traditionally gravitated toward food sources that contain vitamin D, such as the blubber of marine mammals. This trend may have arisen as a way to supplement the diet with vitamin D in the face of inadequate sunlight. Native Americans in Canada and Alaska – who consume less traditional foods than centuries ago – currently have endemic vitamin D deficiency.

So vitamin D is an ancient hormone, preserved through millions of years of evolution. Other animals store vitamin D after either ingesting it or making it through direct exposure to sunlight. All animals, whether or not they spend significant amounts of time in the sun, maintain this hormone system that has its roots in sunlight. However, while it is clear that vitamin D can have an effect on calcium and bones in other animals, the full range functions of vitamin D have not been fully explained. Most of our information on this substance comes from studies of humans, which are the most extensively studied animal on earth.

## 2.3 History of vitamin D in public health

Modern medicine has characterized vitamin D in great detail. We know it is an essential hormone in humans, with many points of action in the body. We know its chemical structure; we can describe where it comes from and how it works on the cell's nucleus. Drug companies tweak its chemical bonds to create new drugs to treat diseases of many organ systems. But the roots of this knowledge, the discovery of vitamin D and its properties, go back to the study of the most extreme form of vitamin D deficiency: the disease called rickets.

The characteristic set of bony deformities of rickets was common in Europe and America during the 1700's and 1800's. During the mid-1900's, rickets was essentially eliminated through public health measures.

However, currently it is returning, and shows up with some regularity in pediatricians' offices and emergency rooms. Its first presentation in an infant, for example, can be new-onset seizures due to low blood calcium levels.

Rickets is a disease of infancy and childhood. Essentially it is the failure of calcium to deposit on the protein scaffolding of the skeleton. In its most extreme form, this lack of calcium leaves a child with characteristic physical signs: the legs are bowed or knock-kneed, the ribs develop a lumpiness, the head is large, the skull is thick, the chest is protruded forward, and the muscles are weak. The child may develop seizures. The skeletal deformities of this disease, left untreated, will persist into adulthood.

Ancient authors in Greece and Rome described this constellation of signs, but it was not studied in detail until the 1600's, when rickets became common. Beginning at this time, industrialization in Northern Europe was pushing the population into cities, where tall buildings cut off sunlight, and pollution and work kept people indoors.

The physician John Mayow, writing in the 1600's,[2] described the syndrome well. This translation from the Latin was published in 1685:

1. *The proportion of the parts is irregular: viz. The Head bigger than it ought to be.*
2. *The Face over-fat.*
3. *The Wit too acute in respect of the Age.*
4. *The external Members, chiefly the musculous, lean and extenuated.*
5. *The Skin loose and flagging.*
6. *The Bones for the most part bowed, and those about the joints standing out, and knotty.*
7. *The Spine or Back-bone is variously inflected.*
8. *The Breast is straight and narrow.*
9. *The Extremities of the Ribs knotty.*

...

*Lastly, to these is added an Enervation of almost all the Parts; also a certain drowsiness and Impatience of Labour and Exercise: For the little Children cannot play, except sitting, and [only] with much ado can stand on their feet. And at last in the Progress of the Disease, the burthen of their Head, can hardly be sustained by their weak neck.*

Mayow ascribed the etiology to an absence of "Animal Spirit" in the body. He felt that nerve tissue carried this substance, and somehow the flow became congealed and sluggish at the base of the brain. In this way, an abundance of "Animal Spirit" in the brain led to a quick and witty disposition, and a lack of it in the body led to weakness and sluggishness. His opinions were not unusual for his day. Francis Glisson, an English physician who described the disease in detail 35 years before Mayow's book was published in English, attributed it to "cold distemper, that is moist and consisting of penury or paucity of and stupefaction of spirits."[3] The physician Daniel Whistler, writing in 1645, noted in rickets an enlargement of the head, of the ends of the long bones and of the abdomen, with "the whole bony system ... flexible like wax that is rather liquid, so that the flabby and toneless legs scarcely sustain the weight of the superimposed body ... they are too feeble to sit up, much less to stand, when the disease is increasing."[4]

Gradually, through application of principles of observation, physicians in the 1800's began to suspect that rickets, like scurvy and beriberi, was a disease of nutrition. In England, the disease was becoming increasingly common, mostly in the cities: dark, overcrowded places. By contrast, the disease was rare in small villages. "Climate has an undoubted influence upon the development of rickets," wrote the French physician Trousseau.[5] "The disease is unquestionably much more common in damp cold countries than elsewhere." Trousseau suggested that absence of sunlight was the cause.

Theobald Palm, an English physician of the late 1800's who had practiced in Japan, noted that rickets was absent in tropical countries.[6] Sunlight, he wrote, "is essential to the healthy nutrition of growing animals ... and is the most important element in the aetiology of the disease." Eventually sunlight was confirmed to treat the disease.

Folk wisdom had long attributed healing powers to cod liver oil, and physicians found that it also prevented and cured rickets. Over the years, cod liver oil became a mainstay of preventive medicine, and many currently living adults remember being lined up in their mothers' kitchens and fed a spoonful of the foul, oily liquid once a day. Incidentally, if one listens to these adults, they frequently will report: "We hated it. But you know, we never got sick."

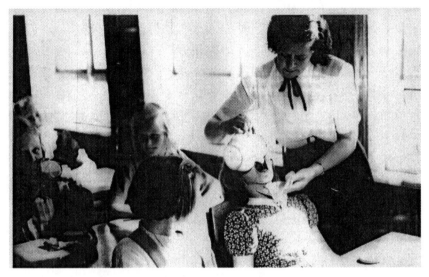

Icelandic children being fed cod liver oil, circa 1940.

Medicine solved the problem of rickets. We learned how to prevent and cure it with a spoonful of fish oil, with which mothers tormented their children for generations.

Later, the public health function of the government became involved. How could one prevent rickets in the entire population? How do you access the people who aren't interested in seeing doctors, or reading newspapers, or learning about the latest in preventive health measures? Just as the government has put chlorine in water to prevent diarrhea deaths, and fluoride in water to prevent cavities, and B-vitamins in flour to prevent nutritional deficiency, it was decided to put vitamin D into the food supply at a dose that would prevent rickets in the average person.

The dosage decided upon was based on cod liver oil. It turned out that one spoonful of the oil contained about 400 units of vitamin D. But how could one get vitamin D into food? Vitamin D is fat soluble – it would be difficult to put it into flour, which contains little fat. Most sources of fat in the diet are not universally eaten in the population, and anyway are not eaten every day.

But milk – that's something that everybody was drinking. And milk contains fat. So the government began requiring that milk distributors add 400 units of vitamin D to an amount of milk that the average person was likely to drink in the average day – one quart.

After this fortification started, rickets all but disappeared in the United States. It stayed in the textbooks, partly for historical purposes, partly to educate students about the function of vitamin D, and partly to educate those health care providers who would care for the most disadvantaged patients. But rickets was more or less lost from medical thinking. Vitamin D deficiency was put in the back of the medical mind; as long as the child was not frankly malnourished, one didn't have to think about it.

Of course, milk has now gone somewhat out of fashion. It certainly is not consumed by the quart in the average household on the average day. And in a predictable fashion, rickets has now reappeared. Children present with seizures to emergency rooms, and are found to have low calcium. They arrive at orthopedists' offices with bowed legs.[7]Rickets has returned. The fortunate part of this story, the kernel of gold inside this dark disease, is that now the issue is once again before us. These children are the alarm bell; they are the canaries in the mine that tell us something is wrong. After all, if a few children are presenting with severe disease, shouldn't there be many, many more children with less severe disease out there in the population, without enough signs and symptoms to prompt physicians to look for vitamin D deficiency? And if it is in children, shouldn't it be in adults, who are subject to the same environmental factors as the children? Shouldn't it be in the mothers who are breastfeeding these infants?

It is likely that as rickets became more common, more subtle forms of vitamin D deficiency began to arise in the urban populations of northern Europe, both in children and in adults. That is, the environmental factors leading to rickets – crowding, living indoors, poor nutrition – affected not only infants and children but individuals of all age in the population, and to varying degrees.

And now that we know that vitamin D isn't really a vitamin at all, but a substance we carry around inside us to compensate for our migration from the tropics, a residue of sunlight – and now that we know that it is really a steroid hormone, one that affects the immune system and the brain and the heart and every organ of the body – shouldn't we be looking for traces of its deficiency in other diseases?

And we must think: should it be left to chance whether people get enough? And is it actually fair that based on things that we can control partly if at all – how far we live from the equator, skin color, how much time we have for exercise outside – is it fair that these things should determine whether the health of individuals is devastated? Is it fair that they should determine, as it clearly does in some cases, whether people live or die?

## 2.4 It's a steroid hormone

When we casually consider the idea of a vitamin deficiency, the ideas that come to mind do not do justice to the magnitude of this problem. The fact that we call this substance "Vitamin D" is unfortunate. To the average person, the word "vitamin" tends to mean a set of desirable but optional additions to our diet that might make us healthier in an auxiliary way. We think of vitamins as present in our food in adequate amounts, and as something consumed in the form of a pill only by those who feel a need for a subjective well-being. Probably this has little or no basis in science, we think. In this case, though, there is a basis in science to think that we can increase our personal well-being through taking a pill containing adequate amounts of this vitamin.

Vitamin D is actually a hormone. It affects every organ in the body. Evolutionarily speaking, we're supposed to be gathering it through routine exposure to the sun. Put another way, the sun regulates all our organ systems through this substance. We're in big trouble without the sun's hormone, and in extreme cases when we're without sun – like most Americans today, living in boxes, hiding from the light – we need to eat a substitute to keep healthy.

Vitamin D falls into a class of hormones called steroids. This group of hormones enters the body's cells, binds to DNA and alters the way it is expressed. DNA is used as the blueprint for manufacturing all the proteins in the body. In this way, steroid hormones, and vitamin D, fundamentally alter the proteins that cells make, and so alter the structure of our bodies.

Please note that the word "steroid" as commonly used in reference to athletic performance enhancement refers to specific subtypes of testosterone only. Vitamin D is not a male hormone. It is similar to the testosterones only in its site of action on the cell's DNA, and in the magnitude of its effect on the body.

The human body produces dozens of different steroid hormones. To examine their extent of influence and varieties of action, let's consider a few.

- Aldosterone is one of the main hormones controlling the body's fluid balance and sodium and potassium content. Deficiency can cause raised potassium and, sometimes, cardiac rhythm disturbances.

- Cortisol is one of the main stress hormones, with a complex set of effects including stress adaptation, blood pressure control, and anti-inflammatory properties. Deficiency of this hormone is life-threatening: the body loses blood pressure and fails to adequately fight simple infections. Varieties of this hormone, including prednisone, are used in medicine to treat inflammation in the body in diseases ranging from arthritis to strep throat.

- Estradiol, the principal estrogen, is produced in the ovaries and causes women to look and behave like women. Estrogen deficiency, such as in women who have had complete hysterectomies before menopause, causes osteoporosis.

- Testosterone, produced in the testicles, makes men look and behave like men, increases muscle and bone mass, and in both sexes stimulates sex drive. Low testosterone levels can cause male infertility.

- Progesterone is an essential hormone in pregnancy, necessary to prepare the uterus for the implantation of the embryo. Without progesterone, pregnancy is impossible.

Imagine that you were without estrogen or testosterone. Would this not have a fundamental impact on your life? Would you be the same person you are now? As you read this, you are likely to be deficient in Vitamin D, another equally powerful, life altering hormone. But what is Vitamin D the hormone of? What body functions are suffering?

Exactly what you are missing has not been described completely by science. We literally do not know what we are missing. However, there are hints in the literature, which will be addressed later in this book.


## 2.5 Vitamin D deficiency currently

In my experience, people with severe vitamin D deficiency have an imploded look. They lack the glow that one expects to see in healthy, active people. Their faces don't shine, they smile less, and their energy is low. They are unhappy, and they have no idea what they are suffering from.   They look outside themselves for the source of their unease, sometimes going to their doctors. Doctors find diseases that circle around the main problem: depression, arthritis, skin disease, or chronic pain, for example. The treatments for these diseases boost the patient's metabolism up a bit, perhaps, or treat some of the pain or some of the discomfort. But this main, underlying steroid hormone deficiency remains.

Vitamin D deficiency can be subtle. There is no red flag that shows up in a doctor's examining room that points toward the diagnosis. It can affect every organ system, probably in ways we have not yet discovered.

As for any disease, though, we need a definition of it to work with. Amongst the wide range of variation in the human population, we need to draw a line, to say, "this is healthy, and this is sick." For vitamin D deficiency, the way medicine has drawn that line is based on the childhood disease rickets. The investigation of rickets led medicine to its first understanding that vitamin D existed, as a hormone that affects calcium and the skeletal system.

I'd like to briefly describe how medicine defines vitamin D deficiency based on its effects on calcium and bone. This definition of the deficiency is based on one organ system only. Vitamin D's effects on other organ systems have not been studied well enough for us to determine how much vitamin D they need to be healthy. So we use the skeletal system as a yardstick, and assume that if it is happy, the rest of the body is likely to be happy, too.

When there isn't enough vitamin D, blood calcium levels tend to drop. Because the body likes to keep calcium levels carefully regulated, another hormone, parathyroid hormone (PTH), becomes increasingly active in an effort to compensate.

Parathyroid hormone is secreted by small, nodular glands located around the thyroid gland in the neck. This hormone causes bone cells called osteoclasts to increase their work of eating away little bits of bone and releasing calcium into the blood circulation. In a healthy person, the activity of osteoclasts balances the activity of cells called osteoblasts, which lay down calcium to make new bone. This constant process of taking apart and rebuilding bone helps keep bones strong. It is as if a bridge made of concrete were being constantly chipped away and re-cemented by construction workers in order to keep it safe.

When PTH levels are elevated, osteoclasts do more work than the osteoblasts – the construction workers are taking apart more of the bridge than they are cementing back together. More calcium is taken up than is laid down, and over the years a thinning of the bones can occur, called osteoporosis. This is one of the ways that vitamin D deficiency leads to osteoporosis.

So given that elevated PTH levels are bad, researchers have defined vitamin D deficiency as the level of vitamin D where PTH starts to increase. This blood level turns out to be somewhere between about 20 and 32 nanograms per deciliter (ng/dL).[8]

In this deficiency state, bone growth is poor, osteoporosis may occur, and blood calcium and phosphate levels may be low. The patient may develop muscle weakness and body-wide pain. Other illnesses also seem to be associated with vitamin D deficiency, but are not considered classic components of the syndrome: defects in the immune system, problems mood and brain function, and heart disease, among others. I discuss these illnesses later in this book.

## 2.5.1 Modern Prevalence

Numerous studies document that vitamin D deficiency is common in many areas of the world. In the following selection of studies, researchers estimated the rate of vitamin D deficiency in various populations using blood levels. The studies had differing definitions of the deficiency; however all were relatively conservative and may underestimate the true extent of the disease.

- In a landmark study published in 1998, 290 consecutive inpatients at a Harvard teaching hospital were tested. 57 percent were vitamin D deficient.[9]
- In France, a study of more than 1,500 people collected from around the country found that at least 14% had vitamin D deficiency. People living in northern areas had a much higher risk.[10]
- In Italy, women attending osteoporosis centers around the nation were studied; at least 76% had low vitamin D levels.[11]
- In a study of low income elderly residents of subsidized housing in Boston, 73% of blacks and 35% of whites had vitamin D deficiency during the wintertime.[12]
- A study of 1248 adolescent girls in Beijing found that 45 percent had vitamin D deficiency during the winter.[13]
- In Iran, a study of 50 mothers at the time of childbirth found that 80 percent had vitamin D deficiency.[14]
- In a study from the Netherlands published in 2006, analysis of blood from new mothers and their children found vitamin D deficiency in 55 percent of immigrant mothers, mostly from Morocco and Turkey, and 54% of these immigrants' babies, based on umbilical cord blood samples. This compares to rates of 5 percent of European descent mothers, and 6 percent of their babies.[15]

This selection of studies on vitamin D deficiency shows the disorder is a worldwide problem. In higher latitudes, relative absence of sunlight is a factor, especially among people with darker pigmentation. In sunnier places, veiling and sheltering from the sun can contribute.

How is one to understand these numbers? A tremendous percentage of the human population is ill with a nutritional deficiency. If it was vitamin C, we would have scurvy everywhere, with bleeding gums and bruising. If it was niacin, we would have an epidemic of skin disease and dementia. If it was iodine, we would see goiters on the necks of one of every three people or so. But what are we seeing now? What is the syndrome of vitamin D deficiency?

Because vitamin D is so fundamental to metabolism, so diverse in its effects on the body, we have not yet described the full spectrum of its deficiency.

## 2.6 Vitamin D in food

It is almost impossible to get enough vitamin D through food. This is a hormone that we should be getting through sun exposure; it is not something that exists in adequate amounts in foods that the average American eats.

For example, in the United States, milk is fortified with vitamin D at 400 units per quart. In order to consume 1,000 units per day – a dose that may not be adequate for good health – one would have to drink 2½ quarts per day. Many Americans do not drink milk, and those who do generally do not drink that amount.

Fish, and especially fish oils, contain significant amounts of vitamin D. Cod liver oil contains about 400 units per teaspoon. However, most people find that drinking a spoonful of fishy, oily liquid once a day is not tolerable. Cod liver oil is available in capsule form, but to get enough one has to consume a great many capsules a day; also, this method is not acceptable for children who cannot swallow pills.

Cod fillets contain about 40 units of vitamin D per four ounce serving. To avoid vitamin D deficiency, you would have to eat several pounds of cod per day. Oily fish tend to have more vitamin D. Canned sardines contain about 240 units and salmon fillets contain about 400 units per four ounce serving. Again, eating adequate amounts of these foods to reach 1,000 units a day is not practical for most people.

Mushrooms contain small amounts of vitamin D. White button mushrooms, the most commonly consumed mushroom in the United

States, have about 20 units per ounce. Preventing vitamin D deficiency with these mushrooms would require consuming about four pounds per day. The chaneterelle variety contains more vitamin D, about 150 units per ounce, but to prevent deficiency one would have to consume at least 6 ounces per day, which would not be practical in most diets.

## 2.7. It's not well studied because of economics

Compared to other substances clamoring for attention in the medical marketplace, vitamin D has a substantial disadvantage. Despite widespread evidence that vitamin D, given orally, might have substantial health benefits on many disease states when given as a drug, pharmaceutical companies are not researching it. The reason is that it is not patentable.

Large drug companies pay for most drug research in the United States. These companies have the potential to invest millions of dollars into drug research and development, but they must be able to recover their investments. For new compounds that the companies develop, patent law allows this recovery to happen. For a number of years after a new drug is put on the market, the company that owns its patent has exclusive rights to its manufacture and sale. The company can price the new drug at any level it chooses, and these pricing levels are chosen to recoup the company's investment and then to make money beyond that amount.

Without patent protection, no company will invest money into researching vitamin D itself. Any money invested in research and development would not be returned, because once vitamin D was discovered to be successful at treating a certain disease, any increase in sales would be enjoyed by all companies making vitamin D, and in fact probably mostly by the company pricing it at the lowest level. Any private company researching naturally occurring vitamin D therefore would be engaging in a self-destructive activity.

However, this is not true if a company can develop a chemical that is similar to vitamin D, but not naturally occurring. Such a compound could be patented, and could therefore be a subject of a drug company's research. And this has in fact happened. Currently, one of the main types of drugs for the skin disease psoriasis is a set of analogs of vitamin D. In psoriasis, the skin develops crusty, flaky patches skin, classically on the elbows and knees. Calcipotriene, sold as a cream under the name Dovonex, is chemically almost identical to vitamin D, but has been adjusted to have less of an effect on blood calcium levels. The way it works is technically unknown, but it clearly decreases the abnormal behavior of skin cells, reducing the proliferation that leads to the skin plaques of psoriasis. Other vitamin D analogs are either on the market currently or under development for use in psoriasis.

While these analogs have received substantial attention from the medical community, there have been very few studies on using the naturally occurring forms of vitamin D in treating psoriasis. Furthermore, psoriasis is typically treated by physicians without evaluating for or treating vitamin D deficiency, which, by the epidemiologic data, must clearly be present in at least a subset of the patients.

Physicians therefore use synthetic analogs of naturally occurring substances rather than the naturally occurring substances themselves to treat psoriasis. If you ask a physician whether they should evaluate for vitamin D deficiency in patients with psoriasis, they will ask you, "Where is the data?" And of course there is little or no data. But we must ask ourselves, why is there no data? And the reason is economic. No one is paying for it.

This is the dilemma facing the nutrition industry. Without patent protection, companies are reluctant to involve themselves in research. But without research, there is no hard evidence for nutrition supplements' effectiveness. This story occurs over and over, and is the main reason why nutritional supplements are controversial. Economic forces act against the investigation and treatment of nutritional diseases.

But there is another way in which the lack of patent protection inhibits the use of vitamin D. Without patent protection, there is no marketing. There are no drug reps going into physicians' offices, buying lunch for the staff, leaving brochures on vitamin D and handing out pens that say, "Remember ergocalciferol for osteoporosis." There are no sophisticated advertising agencies crafting audiovisual messages designed to imprint a message about vitamin D into the conscious and subconscious minds of consumers. Without dramatic messages and aggressive sales tactics, vitamin D cannot compete in today's marketplace of ideas. It doesn't have sexiness; it doesn't have panache. As this is unlikely to change, we are left with making personal decisions based on the available information.

However, it's important to consider the economic aspects of vitamin D from one more point. When we look at the information available, we need to remember that the little bits of it that we have are created despite the economic forces. Very few researchers are creating this information. And so we must avoid a logical fallacy: we must not think that because the evidence is lacking, therefore vitamin D doesn't work or has no significant function. The absence of strong evidence is not the same thing as evidence that vitamin D doesn't work.

## 2.8. Approaching vitamin D decisions

When we read about a health topic, we frequently have an intention to use the information for ourselves or for someone we care about. And indeed as you read this book, I ask that you think about yourself, and your own health risks and problems, and the people you care about.

The world of medicine is complicated and full of unacknowledged uncertainties. Even the guides to it that we may trust – our doctors, our nurses, our therapists – sometimes have contradictory messages and contradictory advice for us. So to at least some extent, we are left thinking about it ourselves, trying on our own to make sense of our options.

Because of the contradictory messages and the complexity of the information available, I advise patients to learn as much as they can about health issues that affect them. In general, the more you know, the more you are likely to make a rational choice about your health.

Now, many people don't want to hear about this. It is difficult to think about disease and one's own mortality. We like to dwell on more happy thoughts. But like some kind of magical spell, thinking about the darker possibilities waiting for us can help us avoid them, and that's another rationale for this intellectual enterprise.

In thinking about our health options, I have found that two things are useful. The first is to be able to understand the medical facts, as they are known. And the second is to have a way to think about them, to turn them over in the mind and apply them to a problem.

Medical facts generally come in the form of published articles in the medical literature. Most patients probably don't have the training or the time to dig through actual medical journal articles, but we do read about the studies, in newspapers, magazines and books. When we do this, it's important to understand a few basics about how the studies are designed, because their design tells us about the reliability of the information we get. In other words, by understanding how studies are put together, we can tell how likely the information they give us is real, and how much might be the static of random information.

Following are main types of medical study. The list is arranged according to the strength of the evidence; study types that are more definitive in their conclusions are at the top:

1.  Randomized controlled trials: In these studies, some patients are assigned randomly to the treatment, and some to a placebo. Preferably, these studies will be "double-blind", meaning that neither the investigators nor the subjects know what the subjects are getting. Having a placebo treatment on a blinded basis means that psychological factors, such as wanting to get better or wanting the treatment to work, can play no role in the outcome. The randomization ensures that the patients in the treatment group will be pretty much the same as the patients in the placebo group.

2.  Cohort studies: These are a type of observational study, meaning that no treatment is assigned to the subjects by the people running the study. Normal medical care is provided. Subjects are enrolled at a point in time and observed, usually for a period of years. Being "observed" might mean only that medical records are reviewed, or it might mean that they drop by a study office a few times a year for some blood tests. Cohort studies can examine a subset of the general population, or can examine people with a specific disease or a

specific exposure, like nuclear plant workers. These studies can give fairly decent information on cause and effect relationships.

3. Case-control studies: This is another type of observational study, though not as strong as a cohort study. Here, people with a disease are examined and compared to people without a disease. The investigators look back in time to figure out what may have happened to them in the past that led to the disease. For example, a case-control study of breast cancer patients might ask women to remember their diet and exercise patterns over the preceding five years. Case-control studies are easier to do and cheaper than cohort studies, and can provide a good first look at a situation before more in-depth investigation is attempted. Public health professionals frequently use the case-control design to investigate disease outbreaks.

4. Case series: This type of study reports a sequence of patients seen by a clinician or a group of clinicians. In general, it is designed to describe what is felt to be a new disease, or to report preliminary results of a new treatment. When used to examine a treatment, this type of study has the disadvantage of having no control arm; one doesn't know whether a treatment described is better than whatever else might have been done.

There are a few other points to consider. First, even if one randomized controlled trial is positive, one shouldn't jump to conclusions. Medical experts generally like to see several randomized controlled trials before concluding that a treatment is effective.

Second, one should be very careful in interpreting information from observational studies, which are frequently reported in the media. Observational studies do not prove that X causes Y – they only show associations. For example, for many years, doctors routinely suggested that women take estrogen supplements after menopause, because observational studies showed that women who took estrogen were much healthier than women who didn't. But after randomized controlled trials were done, it turned out estrogen was not so beneficial.

To see how observational studies can suggest a cause-and-effect relationship where none exists, let's consider an example. Let's say I study pedestrian behavior on city streets, and notice that whenever people open up umbrellas, cars start their windshield wipers. My hypothesis is that the pedestrians are sending a signal to the drivers, who then start their windshield wipers to complete this bizarre ritual.

That's an absolutely wrong conclusion. The rain is causing both of the observed phenomena; they're not causing each other. In the same way, healthy women both took estrogen and had fewer heart attacks.
A third point to consider is the size of the population in the study; the more participants, the more likely the study is to reflect real relationships. Even a randomized controlled trial with a few dozen participants is rather weak.


## 2.8.1 Thinking about vitamin D

When we examine information on health issues, we need to make personal risk-benefit calculations. For vitamin D, there are various risks of the deficiency state. Each of these risks is more or less likely to be real or true. For example, it is clear that having vitamin D deficiency causes osteoporosis, and that it can cause muscle weakness. It is probable that vitamin D deficiency causes a body-wide pain syndrome, though this is perhaps more controversial. And there is evidence to suggest – but it has not been proven – that vitamin D deficiency predisposes one to certain cancers, such as breast and prostate.

The other risk to keep in mind is that of toxicity. What are the risks of taking a certain dose of vitamin D? What is the likelihood that one will experience a side effect? It's a fat-soluble vitamin, so theoretically we need to worry about accumulation.

On the benefit side, we must consider the benefits in terms of convenience of not taking a vitamin supplement every day – it's easier to live one's life without having to remember to take a pill. Also, by not taking a supplement we can be relatively certain we will avoid toxicity of that substance.

But there are also many potential benefits of taking vitamin D supplements: increased energy, increased work performance, better mood, and lower risk of many chronic diseases and cancer. There are varying levels of evidence for all these potential benefits. What I ask you to do is consider the risk of taking 2,000 units of vitamin D per day, as compared to the potential benefits. I believe that the risks are nonexistent, and that the benefits can be tremendous.

*"The light was departing. The brown air drew down*
*All the earth's creatures, calling them to rest*
*From their day-roving, as I, one man alone*

*"Prepared myself to face the double war*
*Of the journey and the pity, which memory*
*Shall here set down, nor hesitate, nor err."*
- Dante, *Inferno*, Canto II, trans. John Ciardi

# 3. Lack of sunlight is related to chronic illnesses

Observational studies have shown that many chronic diseases are more frequent in areas of the world with low sunlight exposure – the higher latitude areas where some humans live. In general, the scientific community does not necessarily attribute these geographical variations directly to vitamin D; it is not clear that vitamin D deficiency causes or helps to cause these diseases. . Instead, the relationship tends to be viewed as a curiosity with many possible explanations that deserve further study. Here are some examples of research findings.

- In a 1990 study, researchers found that the death rate for breast cancer is highest in United States cities with the lowest sun exposure: 17 to 19 deaths per 100,000 women per year in the South and Southwest, versus 33 per 100,000 in the Northeast.[16]
- A 1992 study showed a similar phenomenon for colon cancer: cancer rates were 50 to 80 percent higher in Detroit, Connecticut and Washington state than in New Mexico and Utah.[17]
- In a 1992 study, prostate cancer was shown to be highest in United States counties with the lowest ultraviolet radiation exposure.[18]

- Rates of type 1 or "juvenile" diabetes are up to 10 times higher in countries the farthest from the equator, like Finland, compared to countries that are closer to the equator, like Israel.[19]
- As every medical student is taught, multiple sclerosis, a degenerative neurological disease, is much more common in northern areas of the United States. In a case-control study based on death published in 2000, death from multiple sclerosis was highest in individuals with the lowest estimated exposure to sunlight.[20]
- Schizophrenia, a disease of chronic psychosis, is more common in northern latitudes.[21]

Again, observational studies do not prove causation; they do not prove that low sunlight exposure causes these diseases. However, the associations above do suggest a relationship might exist. As a group, they suggest a single environmental exposure that puts individuals at risk for many chronic diseases. The most likely candidate, in my opinion, is sunlight.

*"[Rickets] is very dangerous and it is totally preventable with vitamin D supplements. These babies fail to thrive, their bones and teeth [become] deformed and they can be in a lot of pain."*
– Dr. Leanne Ward, endocrinologist, Ottawa, Canada.

# 4. Systems and diseases affected by vitamin D

## 4.1 Brain

### 4.1.1 Mood

People get lethargic in the winter. They lose their energy and their edge; they gain weight and like to sleep. It's almost a subtle form of hibernation. Emotionally, about 1 out of 100 people suffer from "seasonal affective disorder" (SAD), a form of mild to moderate depression that varies with the season. SAD affects women more often than men, and is associated with carbohydrate craving and withdrawal from social situations.

It stands to reason that vitamin D, a steroid hormone linked to sunlight exposure, might be linked to seasonal variations in mood. Certainly other steroid hormones affect mood: prednisone, an analog of cortisol, can cause anxiety and even psychosis; birth control pills can cause mood changes; and testosterone replacement in men has been reported to improve subjective well-being. The possibility that vitamin D affects mood has not been well enough studied to draw definitive conclusions. However, two small studies are thought- provoking.

In a 1999 study, researchers at Johns Hopkins University studied 15 people with a diagnosis of SAD.[22] They gave eight subjects a large dose (100,000 units) of vitamin D in a single dose once, and gave seven subjects daily phototherapy – a conventional treatment for seasonal affective disorder involving exposure to a bright, full-spectrum light source – for two hours per day. Both groups received standardized tests for depression before and after the intervention. After one month, the test results for subjects who received the single dose of vitamin D improved; they did not improve for subjects receiving phototherapy. Within the vitamin D group, the more that blood vitamin D levels increased, the better the improvement on the depression scores.

This very small study provides some evidence that vitamin D can improve the symptoms of SAD. Using vitamin D instead of phototherapy would have advantages in cost and convenience over using light therapy.

In another small study conducted during the wintertime in Australia, 44 subjects received either 400 or 800 units of vitamin D or placebo for five days in a randomized, double-blind trial.[23] The subjects were students who were otherwise healthy – no psychiatric illness was present. Subjects receiving vitamin D showed an increase in positive mood compared to those receiving placebo. This is further evidence that vitamin D status is related to mood.

Vitamin D may be related to "major depression," a serious illness that substantially increases risk of suicide. However, this relationship has not been studied formally. Anecdotally, a psychiatrist colleague of mine has reported success in treating several cases of refractory depression by replacing vitamin D. These are people that had been through several trials of different antidepressants.

4.1.2 Schizophrenia
Apart from geography being a risk factor for developing schizophrenia – the farther from the equator, the greater the risk – researchers have found that being born in the wintertime increases the likelihood of developing schizophrenia in later life. During the winter, the mother's vitamin D levels tend to be low, and in some unknown way this seems to affect the fetus's developing brain. The observational data on schizophrenia, combined with some published lab research, has led some epidemiologists and psychiatrists to theorize that vitamin D deficiency in the mother during gestation can predispose an infant to mental illness.[24]

## 4.2 Immune system

Immune cells have receptors for vitamin D, and scientists have demonstrated that vitamin D directly affects these cells. There are epidemiological links between vitamin D status and immune diseases, and vitamin D has been used clinically to help treat them.

Overall, vitamin D seems to affect only one of the two major ways that the immune system kills bad things. The first way, the one that vitamin D does not seem (so far) to affect, is by the production of antibodies, which are large molecules that cling onto bad proteins and cells and mark them for destruction. Other cells then come along and eat them up. This is the way the body fights most bacterial infections. As a sort of side effect, antibodies also provide a handy tool for diagnosis. If we suspect a certain disease, frequently we can run a blood test for antibodies that gives us a clue in the diagnostic reasoning process.

The second way the immune system works is through cells that directly kill hostile cells and bacteria. This second kind of immune reaction is called "cell-mediated immunity," and it seems to be the system that vitamin D affects. Cell-mediated immunity involves a subset of white blood cells called T lymphocytes. These cells patrol the body for cells that don't look right – cells that seem to be infected by a virus or parasite, or cells that have cancer-like characteristics. When a T cell finds a cell like this, it kills it. In this way, despite the immediate sacrifice of a cell, the potential damage to the body as a whole is minimized.

Vitamin D's relationship to T cell immunity seems to be educational, in a way. Vitamin D helps T cells avoid attacking things they shouldn't be attacking; it helps them know which things are parts of the body that should be left alone. Another way of putting this is that vitamin D helps prevent autoimmune diseases – diseases in which the body, in a fit of irrational exuberance, attacks itself. Vitamin D seems to be necessary in order to keep the immune system in check, to keep it from responding excessively to things it shouldn't bother with. Examples of autoimmune diseases linked to vitamin D are type 1 diabetes, or what used to be called juvenile diabetes; rheumatoid arthritis; and multiple sclerosis.

### 4.2.1 Type 1 diabetes mellitus

In type 1 diabetes, T cells get overly exuberant and attack the cells in the pancreas that make and secrete insulin, the beta cells. Insulin is the hormone that keeps blood glucose levels from rising above a healthy level, and allows the body's tissues to take up and use glucose. Without insulin, blood sugar levels rise. In the short term, blood sugars that rise enough can cause coma. In the long term, high sugars cause widespread tissue damage in the body, and put patients at risk of heart disease, kidney failure and blindness, among other diseases. Classically, type 1 diabetes is a disease of children, but it can occur in patients in their 30's and 40's as well. People with type 1 diabetes tend to die young.

The incidence of type 1 diabetes varies by geography; the disease becomes more common farther from the equator. This suggests that sunlight might play some kind of role in the origin of the disease. Epidemiological researchers also have found that the risk of childhood diabetes seems to be decreased if a child is given vitamin D supplements during the first year of life, and if the child's mother took cod liver oil, a good source of vitamin D, during pregnancy.[25]

Apart from the epidemiologic evidence, researchers have found a vitamin D link while working with a special strain of mouse that is susceptible to type 1 diabetes, the "non-obese diabetic" (NOD) mouse. This mouse is commonly used as a model to study the characteristics and therapy of the disease. In one study, injecting these mice with active vitamin D prevented inflammation of the pancreas in every mouse that received it.[26]

### 4.2.2 Rheumatoid arthritis

Rheumatoid arthritis is an autoimmune disease in which the body attacks its own joints. Patients have a painful swelling that tends to appear in the body symmetrically: for example, the small bones of the hand might be affected on both sides of the body. Apart from affecting joints, patients with rheumatoid arthritis can also have some autoimmune spillover into other organ systems, including anemia, and various disorders of the eye and lung.

Analyzing data from more than 40,000 women enrolled in the Iowa Women's Health Study – a cohort study – researchers found that women who had the highest consumption of vitamin D, either through food or through supplements, had about a 30 percent lower risk of eventually developing rheumatoid arthritis compared to women with the lowest vitamin D intake.[27]

In one small, uncontrolled study, researchers found that an analog of active vitamin D, alphacalcidiol, when given over a three-month period reduced the severity of rheumatoid arthritis in 17 of 19 patients.[28] Nine patients actually went into complete remission. Of course one has to worry about elevated blood calcium levels with active vitamin D. However, no patients had elevated blood calcium. Six patients had to have their active vitamin D doses reduced after they developed high urine levels of calcium. As of this writing, alphacalcidiol was not available for prescription use in the United States.

### 4.2.3 Lupus

There is some evidence that the autoimmune disease lupus has a vitamin D link. Lupus, like rheumatoid arthritis, attacks the joints, but is more predisposed to attack multiple organ systems. Commonly involved components of the disease are rash, arthritis, kidney disease, anemia and disorders of the brain including psychosis and seizures. Lupus has a geographic distribution that suggests it has a sunlight component. It is classically a disease of women of childbearing age, particularly African-American women, but it can affect all sexes, races and ages. Vitamin D levels in patients with lupus have not been extensively studied, but a few researchers have found high rates of vitamin D deficiency in lupus patients. [29]

### 4.2.4 Multiple Sclerosis

Multiple sclerosis, another autoimmune disease with a sunlight-deprived geographic pattern, affects the brain. White blood cells attack the coating of nerve cells, causing a wide range of neurologic symptoms. These can include confusion, an inability to move smoothly, weakness, paralysis and blindness. This is usually a disease of adulthood. It can be a rapid and devastating disease in certain patients, however in general it shortens life expectancy by about seven years.

There is some evidence from animal experiments that vitamin D might be involved in the onset of multiple sclerosis, and that it might help with treatment.

The strongest study involving humans, though, involves prospective observational data from the Nurses' Health Study and the Nurses' Health Study II, cohort studies which followed women for 10 to 20 years.[30] Women who ingested the highest amount of vitamin D were 33 percent less likely to develop MS than women who ingested the least. The strength of this study comes from the large number of subjects, and the fact that it was prospective, following them over time rather than looking backward. Still, there is a chance for error here, because there were no randomization, controls or blinding, as in a clinical trial.

As of this writing, there is little direct evidence that vitamin D will treat multiple sclerosis. However, it might. And certainly it makes sense to treat the glaring, underlying nutritional deficiency that many patients with multiple sclerosis have.

### 4.3 Cancer

Vitamin D seems to have a normalizing effect on cells. As tissues grow and repair themselves, cells have less of a tendency to more into an aggressively growing mode, and are more likely to grow into what they should be, if under the influence of adequate vitamin D.

Observational data shows links between vitamin D and cancer risk for colon, breast, ovarian and prostate cancer.

For example, a study based on data from the Center for Disease Control and Prevention (CDC) has indicated that vitamin D intake reduces breast cancer risk.[31] Every decade or so, the CDC interviews and examines a cross-sectional sample of the US population in a program called the National Health and Nutrition Examination and Survey (NHANES). Huge amounts of data are collected, organized, stripped of information that might compromise an individual's confidentiality, and made available publicly for whoever would like to analyze them. In one such analysis, researchers compared women with breast cancer to women without breast cancer. They found that sunlight exposure and vitamin D intake were lower in the women with breast cancer.

Researchers actually are investigating vitamin D as a treatment for prostate cancer. Calcitriol, a form of activated vitamin D widely used to treat patients with renal failure, is being examined in combination with a the chemotherapeutic agent docetaxel in a multicenter trial. Early results are promising.[32]

## 4.4 Bone

The story of osteoporosis and its treatment in America is an example of perverse incentives in the medical marketplace. Osteoporosis is on the rise, we are told, and the right thing to do is to take the expensive, patented drugs to stop it – and if we can catch it early, all the better. But I have found that few clinicians evaluate patients with osteoporosis for the most common known cause of "secondary" osteoporosis, vitamin D deficiency.

Vitamin D hasn't been explored as a drug for the treatment of osteoporosis, and it may never be as long as medical research funding continues in its current pattern. It is, in my opinion, probable that ergocalciferol 50,000 units per week is as safe and effective as one of the newer drugs, but we do not know currently. Typically doctors will put people on vitamin D, to be sure, but at a dose far lower than what is probably necessary even to maintain vitamin D status at a low level in the body, much less to replace it to physiologic levels.

## 4.5 Muscle Strength

The exact strength of your legs may not be a concern to you if you are young, healthy and not an athlete. Older adults, however, tend to suffer a progressive loss of leg strength with age, to the point where climbing stairs and getting into and out of a car can be difficult by the time one reaches 70 years or so. This phenomenon usually does not ring alarm bells from a medical point of view, other than denoting an increased risk of falls and a need for exercise. With low vitamin D levels, though, muscles become inflamed and weak. This is one variety of the large category muscle diseases, or myopathies.

In vitamin D deficiency, the proximal muscles of the body are strongly affected: the larger muscles closest to the center of the body, that is, the thigh and upper arm muscles. As these muscles weaken, activities that require lifting the arm and leg become difficult. As the myopathy progresses, the patient is not able to rise from a chair, and becomes dependent on a wheelchair. The weakness may be attributed to nerve degeneration such as occurs in diabetes, to general ill health, or to the "dwindles" of old age.

However, when vitamin D deficiency is causing such weakness, the disorder is easily treatable. Vitamin D supplementation rapidly reduces inflammation and muscle weakness, and restores muscle strength. People formerly confined to wheelchairs can stand up again.

This sounds dramatic. In fact, the idea of people standing up from wheelchairs brings up images of faith-healing church services of dubious authenticity. But this is not a miracle. It is simply the correction of a chronic nutritional deficiency.

A series of five weak, wheelchair-bound patients successfully treated with vitamin D supplementation was described by a group of endocrinologists in Buffalo in the April 24, 2000 issue of *Archives of Internal Medicine.*[33] After vitamin D replacement, four of the five could walk without support, and the fifth could walk with support. Interestingly, the four patients who did the best also were subsequently free of the body-wide aches and pains that they had been experiencing for years.

An example was a 37-year-old African American female with severe, longstanding diabetes. She had had aches and pains and weakness for several months. She had trouble combing her hair, an activity that uses the proximal muscles of the arm, and was unable to walk. Vitamin D (as ergocalciferol) 50,000 units once per week for six weeks eliminated her symptoms.

These anecdotes are examples of a generally medically accepted phenomenon of myopathy due to vitamin D deficiency. However, they are extreme cases. Can vitamin D help people with less pronounced weakness?

In a ranomized controlled trial published in the Journal of the American Geriatrics Society, elderly residents of assisted living facilities and nursing homes had about 30 percent fewer falls if they received 1,000 units of vitamin D daily.[34]

The overall picture is of an endemic nutritional deficiency that can, in its most severe form, cause profound weakness and immobility. It is probably open to question whether mild deficiency causes a more subtle disability.

But even by a conservative estimate of the prevalence of this problem worldwide, it is a tragedy that there may be thousands of immobile, elderly people in nursing homes that could benefit from this simple intervention.

### 4.6 Pain

Physicians find it difficult to treat patients who say, "my whole body hurts." Such a description doesn't fit into the standard medical model for understanding pain, and such complaints occasionally are attributed to a psychiatric problem. However, body-wide pain can be a symptom of vitamin D deficiency. This syndrome is well documented in the medical literature.

The patient will experience deep, bony or muscle pain that may focus on the legs, especially the shins, but can affect any part of or the entire body. Occasionally the patient will experience an extreme tenderness of the skin, such that even light pressure to the forearms causes pain. In a study from the Mayo Clinic, even patients taking vitamin D supplements were susceptible to this syndrome; apparently the supplements were not adequate to keep blood vitamin D levels high enough.[35]

This syndrome may be distinct from fibromyalgia; the Mayo Clinic study excluded patients with this diagnosis. However, vitamin D levels in fibromyalgia have not been well studied, and low levels may play a part in it, as well. In this study, the pain syndrome occurred in all ethnic groups and at all ages. It should be noted that the Mayo Clinic is located in Minnesota, a northern location where ambient light is reduced through much of the year.

The reasons that vitamin D deficiency causes this unusual pain syndrome are unclear. Dr. Michael Holick of Boston University, a vitamin D researcher, theorizes that when vitamin D levels drop, bone cells called osteoblasts continue to lay down the protein infrastructure of bone, even when calcium and phosphate levels are not high enough for good bone formation.[36] The proteins then become soggy with water, which puts pressure on the lining of bones, which in turn causes pain. The muscle pains of vitamin D deficiency may be due to the myopathy that the deficiency induces. Other features of this pain disorder are unexplained, however; for example it is unclear how vitamin D deficiency might cause extreme skin tenderness.

Vitamin D may also play a part in more typical types of pain. In a study published in the journal *Spine*, researchers found vitamin D deficiency in 83 percent of patients complaining of low back pain at a clinic in Saudi Arabia.[37] While this study had no controls, the authors state that vitamin D therapy decreased pain in all patients with the deficiency.

## 4.7 Skin

In the skin, vitamin D acts in a "differentiation" mode to encourage skin cells to develop in a normal way. This action is evident in the disease psoriasis.

Psoriasis is a chronic disease in which patches of skin become inflamed and red, and can develop a silvery crust. The lesions tend to appear on the knees and elbows, but they can affect any part of the body, including the scalp, causing a form of dandruff. Essentially the skin cells become exuberant; they become excessively enthusiastic and make extra skin cells that then accumulate and flake off the body in chunks.

Researchers have found that giving active vitamin D either orally, or topically as a cream, effectively treats psoriasis. In fact, vitamin D analogs currently are one of the primary modes of treating psoriasis. Note that the reason for using analogs is partly due to the fact that naturally occurring vitamin D is not patentable, and so for-profit drug companies do not seek to make products of it, as discussed above.

Another standard treatment for psoriasis is ultraviolet light therapy, given by a physician. Ultraviolet light makes vitamin D in the skin, and vitamin D may be part of the mechanism by which ultraviolet light is effective. Interestingly, many patients report that sunlight decreases the severity of their disease.

So given that psoriasis is improved by ultraviolet light, and because the only natural way to get ultraviolet light is from sunlight, the skin seems to need some sunlight in order to be healthy, at least in some people. This is in contradiction to current recommendations from dermatologists, who have been recommending an absolute minimization of sun exposure to reduce risk of skin cancer. It's not clear what the exact truth will be when the battle is over between these two lines of reasoning.

## 4.8 Heart

Vitamin D is related to blood pressure. Studies have found that the higher a person's level of 1,25 vitamin D (the active form of the vitamin), the lower their blood pressure. These studies do not prove that vitamin D deficiency causes high blood pressure, but it is suggestive.

Vitamin D suppresses the activity of the renin-angiotensin-aldosterone hormone system, which is one of the main regulators of blood pressure.[38] The most recent classes of medications that affect this system are called the angiotensin converting enzyme inhibitors, or ACE inhibitors, and angiotensin receptor blockers, or ARBs. Apart from controlling blood pressure, these medications are very effective at reducing death rates from congestive heart failure, a syndrome that occurs when a weakened heart cannot effectively pump blood.

ACE inhibitors and ARBs are examples of drugs that may be working downstream from where the real problem is in many patients. If vitamin D proves to be an effective blood pressure reducing agent – and it hasn't been studied – then it may be that vitamin D deficiency is the primary cause of some cases of high blood pressure. Using ACE inhibitors and ARBs would then be treating the symptoms and not the disease.

If this is true, if vitamin D deficiency can cause hypertension, it might explain the high rates of hypertension in African Americans, who tend to have lower vitamin D levels than individuals of other races and ethnicities.

Please note that you should not stop taking any blood pressure medications after reading this.

### 4.9 Obesity

Observational data indicate there is a relationship between obesity and vitamin D deficiency. A cohort study in Norway from 1994 found that men and women who consumed the least vitamin D were more likely to be obese.[39] In another study, researchers found that among healthy women, obesity was related to lower blood vitamin D levels.[40] This may be because vitamin D spreads out in the body through fatty tissues, and having more fat lowers the concentration of vitamin D through dilution. It is not clear whether increasing one's vitamin D intake will reduce weight.

### 4.10 Height

Vitamin D affects how tall one grows to be by affecting the strength and growth of bones. This is at least evident in the disease rickets: people with the disease are short, and have bowed legs. But just like any other disease, rickets probably has a spectrum that extends into what we call "normal". There are probably millions of Americans whose height is shorter than it could be due to a relatively mild childhood vitamin D deficiency.

In fact, when I look at the shins of my friends and patients – you should try this – I notice that tall individuals have straight shins, and shorter ones have curved shins, in the manner of rickets. This is something that has not been examined in the scientific literature, as far as I can determine.

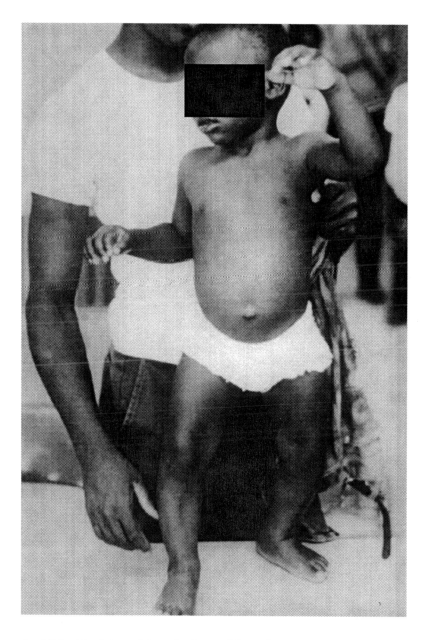

A child with rickets. Note the bowed legs. Source: Centers for Disease Control and Prevention.

*"... A Dungeon horrible, on all sides round*
*As one great Furnace flam'd, yet from those flames*
*No light, but rather darkness visible*
*Serv'd only to discover sights of woe,*
*Regions of sorrow, doleful shades, where peace*
*And rest can never dwell, hope never comes*
*That comes to all; but torture without end*
*Still urges, and a fiery Deluge, fed*
*With ever-burning Sulphur unconsum'd:*
*Such place Eternal Justice had prepar'd*
*For those rebellious, here their Prison ordain'd*
*In utter darkness ..."*
- John Milton, *Paradise Lost*

# 5. Phenomenology: what vitamin D deficiency feels like

Perhaps the best summary of the subjective effects of vitamin D was Dr. Mayow's, from more than 300 years ago: it replenishes one with the "animal spirit," the essence of life, a movement toward what is light and good. Just as microscopic ocean creatures respond to the sun by increasing activity, so we become awakened, alert and active when we are exposed to this steroid hormone.

In the light, we are active, optimistic, and purposeful. In the darkness, something else happens. In Western culture, we associate darkness with Hell, with hopelessness, with loss and solitude. Madness is a kind of darkness of the soul, we tend to think, and that is part of the shame of mental illness. Darkness brings death, and poetically, death is a darkness that we must all pass into. Darkness also can describe the time that we spend waiting for inspiration; the dark night of the soul precedes the apprehension of God's presence.

Light, on the other hand, is the realm of angels, of life, of beauty and truth. Light shows us the way, brings us peace, and settles our souls. The sunflower turns toward the light, and we, if we have made moral choices and live a good life, gladly turn toward the light as well.

This is some of the poetic thinking that underlies our European languages. This thinking underlies our thoughts, and a subconscious version of these thoughts informs our instincts.

These thoughts center on the idea that the light is a blessing, something given to us that perhaps we do not deserve. It is something that we are separated from, and something that we are in danger of being eternally separated from.

And in fact, in the history of much of Europe and the United States, we literally are separated from the light. For much of the year, the sun is low on the horizon. In the fall, we and our ancestors have watched its zenith sink daily, weakening. We track it with astronomy and stone monuments, hoping in some way, but mostly knowing, that it will come back and bless us again.

Is it just the stimulation to our eyes that we miss, and is it only the fertility of the land that is the focus of our anxiety?

Clearly the answer is no. The sun reaches directly into our bodies; it is part of the biochemical structure of our lives. We literally need it to live. The light must touch us, or else we must reach out through the food chain to something the light does touch. If we don't have this, we get sick and then we die. This is plain scientific fact.

As we watch the sun retreat, our strength retreats; our "animal spirit" goes into hibernation. As the darkness settles in, we are left with a residue of what made us strong, and as we face the darkness, that residue diminishes; we dwindle away, and become one with the darkness.

The people living in darkness do not know they are in darkness. They have no conception of what they are missing. They may feel sick, yes; but the doctor says there is nothing wrong. Or perhaps the doctor says that they have depression, or thyroid disease. Later, the doctor may say they have something more serious, like lupus. "Why do I have this disease?" they ask, and we answer, "It's an immune disease," or, "It's just something you can get when you're older," or, "It's genetic."

Perhaps the person in darkness looks at a relative retiring in Florida, or someone from the old neighborhood who is now happy, walking the beach, fishing, smiling more, and walking taller. And the person living in darkness wants to move there too. They may even know that it is the light they want – but it can't really be the light, can it? That's just psychological, they think. It's warmer down there, that's what it is.

But it is the light that makes the difference.

Those without the light break my heart. I see them implode, faces becoming dull, eyes losing a sharpness, skin lacking a healthy glow. They become tired, they ache. They become depressed, moody, paranoid. Starting in October or November, the disease spreads. In the supermarket, on the street, in the hospital: everyone has the dullness, the torpor, the pain. They become fatalistic: this is what life is, they think. This is how it has to be. This is what God has given us, they may say, and we will live with this.

But we don't have to live like this. There is an antidote to the darkness, and it is simple. The antidote to the darkness is to reach out for the traces of the light, for the biochemical trace that the light leaves in us.

A fire heats our home, the trucks bring the fruit from distant farms, phones let us talk to our friends in distant places – and one chemical lets us touch and gain strength from the sun. It is the humble, easy to ignore, almost laughably-named substance called vitamin D.

*"The recommendations of the Food and Nutrition Board with respect to oral vitamin D input fall into a curious zone between irrelevance and inadequacy. For those persons with extensive solar exposure, the recommended inputs add little to their usual daily production, and for those with no exposure, the recommended doses are insufficient to ensure desired 25(OH)D concentration."*

    – John Jacob Cannell, MD, Executive Director, Vitamin D Council

# 6. Stories from patients

- Sarah, a 59-year-old African-American nurse who had no psychiatric diagnosis, started taking 2,000 units of vitamin D a day in the fall of 2003: "Before I started taking it, I would feel tired and sluggish, especially in the morning when I got out of bed for work. And then after I started taking it, I had more energy when I got off of work, and more energy when I got up. And I think even my stamina was better, because I run around here all day." Sara says she felt the quality of her sleep was better. "Maybe because you're more rested, you're more tolerant to things, to the pace, to the chaos. You're more tolerant to chaotic situations."

- Jim, a middle-aged male: "I used to come home from work whipped and semi - catatonic. I would eat, sit around and mope, sleep and go to work again. Given my general fatalist pessimism mixed in with this, it was like living death." Then he started taking 1,200 units of vitamin D a day, with a multivitamin. "Within a couple of weeks, I had more energy, many aches and pains in my bones and joints had receded, and I came somewhat out of my slough of despondency. I'm still not the dancing in the streets type. But the point is that I was able to do other things than work. I don't know if it's a placebo effect, but so far, it's helping."

- An 80-year-old man had a body-wide skin rash, extremely itchy, that had persisted for more than 10 years. Multiple dermatologists had failed to correct the problem. After reading one of my columns on vitamin D, he started taking 1,000 units per day. The rash disappeared.

- A 40-year-old woman who had been on disability due to depression and chronic fatigue was diagnosed with vitamin D deficiency. She received 50,000 units of ergocalciferol, once per week for eight weeks. At the end of the course she said, "I've never felt so good in my life. Give me more."

- A 45-year-old nurse with asthma, initially skeptical about the benefit of a nutritional supplement, was able to stop using two of her three inhaled medications after starting vitamin D.

- My mother, a 65-year-old nurse, had vitamin D deficiency. I saw her in the winter of 2003 and she had that imploded, chronically ill, listless look. She told me that she had had chronic muscle pain for years, and now it was basically intolerable. "The whole thing has been developing gradually over a long period of time, I'd say 20 years. It's very insidious. I would have periods of time when I would ache all over. I remember hearing about fibromyalgia in 1980 when I thought, I bet I have that, because I ache all the time. ... It just gradually got worse. It's been particularly worse over the last 7 or 8 years. The soreness seemed to be around my ligaments. It did not feel like arthritis – it felt like it was in the tissues surrounding the joints. I remember saying, 'I can't believe this is normal. I hurt too much.' ... Within the last year, it was getting worse. It was very, very difficult to get up if I was on the floor. Now that I'm stronger [after vitamin D replacement] I note the difference." On that winter day in 2003, I gave her one capsule containing 50,000 units of vitamin D – a prescription form – and she felt substantially better in two days. She now takes over the counter vitamin D, but she asks me for more of the prescription strength supplement whenever I see her.

*"What is laughter, what is joy, when the world is ever burning? Shrouded by darkness, would you not seek the light?"*
- Dhammapada

# 7. Interviews with vitamin D researchers

In 2005, I called several prominent vitamin D researchers to get their informal perspectives on the problem. Following are notes from those conversations.

Reinhold Vieth, Ph.D., is an associate professor at the University of Toronto and an author of more than 40 scientific papers on vitamin D.

"We evolved as naked apes at equatorial latitudes," Vieth said. "No matter what your skin color, a day out in the sun" – exposing most of your skin – "will generate easily 10,000 units of vitamin D." That figure far exceeds to the current average oral intake of vitamin D of about 200 units per day, Vieth said. "My working theory is that 4,000 units is essentially a level that would match at least the Paleolithic intakes.

"The case is well made; the problem is implementation. It's a matter of convincing people. My feeling is that at least for adults, they should change the RDA up to 2,000 units a day. Once your multivitamins and quart of milk all have 2,000 units, then what we're discussing is moot." For any individual, the health effects of such a change potentially would be equal to quitting smoking, Vieth said.

Sunlight and oral intake in vitamin form should be roughly equivalent, Vieth said. "I don't think there's any reason that sunshine would be advantageous over vitamin D supplementation."

"The reason it's exciting is that it opens a kind of magic box" of possible health effects, he said. "There's not a downside, because the target levels that I describe are biologically natural for the human species." But, for some reason, "people are phobic of it."

Robert Heaney, MD is an osteoporosis researcher at Creighton University Medical Center in Omaha, Nebraska.

"There is a chance that this may be one of the biggest items in all of the recent history of public health – but just a chance.

"It's a bit like trying to figure out what the cause of lung cancer is when everybody smokes. It could well be that because deficiency is nearly uniform, that we may have overlooked its role in a dozen or more chronic disorders, ranging from cancer to multiple sclerosis.

"That's one possible outcome of all this. The other extreme is that it's going to be like all of these other things that flash large on the radar screen, and then shrink back down and assume a small but significant role. I don't know where it's going to come down – somewhere along that spectrum."

The common perception of vitamin D toxicity in the nutrition and medical communities is exaggerated, he said. "I've done several studies using 10,000 units a day with no evidence of toxicity, but I don't think it's necessary to use that much." Even after five months, there were no cases of high calcium levels in the blood or urine, which would be the earliest signs of toxicity.

"The curious thing is that we did this with a group of African Americans this past year, and many of them volunteered that they felt better than they had in years and had fewer aches and pains, which we didn't even ask about."

Research on vitamin D is limited due to lack of funding. "There's no money in it. The NIH peer review process doesn't look on nutrition as really science and they don't like to fund it. And there's no money in the supplement industry. Vitamin D is dirt-cheap. There is no industry money going into it, and no government money going into it."

Bess Dawson-Hughes, MD, professor of Medicine at Tufts University, has published more than 40 scientific articles on vitamin D.

Dawson-Hughes said that the medical community increasingly is accepting the benefits of vitamin D. "It's changing pretty significantly, because the evidence is mounting at a fairly rapid clip. The evidence really has to drive the situation, and it is starting to do so." However, "I think people resist it on principle. They feel like, how could a deficiency be so prevalent?"

The elderly in particular have a very high prevalence of vitamin D deficiency, and because of that many have decreased muscle strength. Dawson-Hughes's research has found that elderly people with low vitamin D levels are slower to stand from a chair, and walk more slowly than those with higher levels. Furthermore, prospective, randomized trials have shown that elderly people who take vitamin D seem to have a lower overall risk of falling – about 22 percent less than those who take placebo, she said.

Dawson-Hughes said that the increase in muscle strength that comes with good vitamin D levels is continuous – the higher the level, the more muscle strength there is. To put it another way, "I don't think you have to be profoundly vitamin D deficient to have some level of impairment in muscle performance," she said. "I think we need to rethink what the optimal level, what the goal line should be.

"Food fortification or supplement use in these northerly latitudes is really going to have to come into wider use. Sun exposure in the summertime will do the job, but there's a lot of negativity toward that in the dermatology community. ... A lot of the elderly just don't get sun exposure. They're not outside, and they're wearing hats, and they're concerned about getting another skin cancer."

Even if they do get sun in the summertime, "it would not tide them over the winter. A wintertime solution has to be found. I think for simplicity sake, boosting the oral take is the most feasible approach."

John Jacob Cannell, MD, executive director of The Vitamin D Council, is a psychiatrist and vitamin D researcher at Atascadero State Hospital in California.

"I think this problem is perhaps only second to smoking as the most important public health problem in the United States," Cannell said.

Cannell's moment of insight came when he learned that humans living in full tropical sunlight make 10,000 to 20,000 units of vitamin D per day in their skin. "It changed my life," he said. "When I read that fact it shook me. Nature would never have made that system unless there was a reason for it.

"I'm not really a health food nut – I don't believe that vitamin C cures cancer. But if you talk about vitamin D the question is, is 10,000 units per day better than 400? The fact that you make so much, so quickly, the fact that we have migrated from Africa – we're conducting a large experiment. Let's take the most potent steroid in the human body out of humans to see what happens.

"The mistake by the government is so huge."

Cannell has noticed that patients who receive vitamin D supplementation have an improvement in mood. "Some patients have a reduction in hypertension. I've seen patients with type 2 diabetes with strong improvement, some getting off their oral meds."

The government has tremendously overestimated vitamin D's toxicity, he said.

"The government says 2,000 units per day is safe for everybody. But in reality you can take 10,000 units per day and it won't hurt you."

Bruce Hollis, Ph.D. is a researcher in the departments of Pediatrics and of Biochemistry and Molecular Biology at the Medical University of South Carolina.

"Many vitamins you can get from your food," he said. "Unfortunately, vitamin D isn't one of them.

"Basically, it doesn't occur in food. But it was never meant to be taken in food to begin with. It was meant to be gotten from sun exposure, and until the last few centuries, we got plenty of it. You have a unique case here."

The public health community will be slower to educate the public about this problem than physicians can be, Hollis said. "The physician needs to educate the people about this. But the physician looks at this as thrown together with all the other vitamins – it's like Linus Pauling standing on the street corner screaming about vitamin C. But this isn't like that. This is a big problem that cannot be solved by conventional means."

Sunlight is probably not a viable option for most people, Hollis said. For example, African Americans with darker pigment have to spend about an hour and a half per day in the sun to maximize their vitamin D production for the day. "People don't have the time, and a lot of times it's uncomfortable.

"So the physician has to treat with a prescription drug, or you're going to have to change the RDA guidelines. I think a realistic amount is probably in the 2,000-unit range, depending on the situation. It's not one dose fits all. The last guideline said that 2,000 units was the upper safe intake, and that's totally wrong. It's many thousands." You would have to take 50,000 units of vitamin D a day for many days to reach a toxic state, he said.

The laboratory range for "normal" vitamin D levels traditionally has been established by measuring levels in large populations, and calling the middle 96 percent of that range "normal".

"What if they took a bunch of women, and half were post-menopausal, and they plotted estrogen, and said this is normal? It makes no sense physiologically," Hollis said. In other words, what a lab calls "normal" may not be healthy.

Another misconception about vitamin D is that because it is fat-soluble, it must be stored in the fat. "Vitamin D really isn't stored in the fat," Hollis said. "It's basically stored in extracellular fluid.

"As soon as you stop taking vitamin D, your plasma levels go off the cliff. If it was fat storage, you'd see a slow release back into the circulation. It's not there."

*"Throughout my preparation of this review, I was amazed at the lack of evidence supporting statements about the toxicity of moderate doses of vitamin D. Consistently, literature citations to support them have been either inappropriate or without substance."*

–   Dr. Reinhold Vieth, writing on the toxicity of vitamin D, in an academic review article.

## 8. Vitamin D is toxic in very high doses

The idea of taking a vitamin D supplement frightens some people because it is a fat-soluble vitamin. Fat-soluble vitamins, we are told, easily accumulate to toxic levels in the body. And it is true that vitamin D can reach toxic levels in the body. However, the dose required to reach toxic levels is far beyond what it is possible to consume without abusing prescription medicines.

Let's look at an example of actual vitamin D toxicity to get a sense of what it is necessary to consume in order to become toxic from this substance.

In Massachusetts during the late 1980's and early 1990's, public health officials investigated a home-delivery dairy that turned out to be over-fortifying their milk with vitamin D. Apparently the equipment that measured vitamin D concentrations was broken, and dairy workers were adding the supplement to the milk without measuring it. Health officials found that the vitamin D content of the milk was 70 to 600 times the legal limit of 500 units per quart set by state law. That works out to 35,000 to 300,000 units per quart in the over-fortified milk.

Over six years of over-fortification, there was very little hint of a problem with vitamin D toxicity among the 11,000 households served by the dairy. Investigators eventually found only 19 people who had illnesses related to the vitamin D. That works out to about 1 case per 10,000 persons per year.

So let's put that into perspective. Let's say each person was drinking 8 ounces of milk per day, and we'll say that the average vitamin D fortification level was only 35,000 units – the lowest level found in the samples the government took. So based on those numbers, in order to get a very low rate of vitamin D toxicity, you have to give people at least – and probably much more than – 8,750 units per day over the course of years. That dosage is 12 times the current USRDA for elderly people.

Now even if we were going to be paranoid and borderline unreasonable, we still could say that it is safe to take 2,000 units per day orally, because there is absolutely no evidence – not even bad, circumstantial, unverified or really old evidence – to indicate that this can be toxic. Probably it's safe to take more, but let's not push it that far. Let's continue to be paranoid. As paranoiacs, we can say with certainty that 2,000 units per day is safe.

*"I love Bosco, it's rich and chocolatey.*
*Chocolate-flavored Bosco is mighty good for me.*
*Mama puts it in my milk for extra energy.*
*Bosco gives me iron and sunshine Vitamin D.*
*Oh, I love Bosco, that's the drink for me."*
  - Television commercial, circa 1950.

# 9. Getting enough vitamin D

The standard way for most land animals to get vitamin D seems to be through direct exposure to sunlight. We, as apes of African-origin, fall into that category. In the millions of years of evolution during which we became human, we were outdoors, living and working in the sun for many hours on the average day. As modern humans settled into various habitats throughout the world, skin pigment evolved in a way to balance out the harmful and beneficial effects of the sun, so that we could make enough vitamin D while not getting skin cancer. Tropical dwelling humans developed dark skin, and the ones exposed to less light developed lighter skin.

Today, humans living in industrialized economies tend to spend most of their time indoors. We have become very aware of the damaging effects of the sun's ultraviolet radiation, and when we go outside we sometimes put chemicals on our skin – sun block – to prevent sunburn and to reduce our risk of cancer in the long term.

These days, if we choose to collect vitamin D through direct sun exposure, we are running a risk – we really don't know where the balancing point is between getting enough sun exposure to avoid vitamin D deficiency, and getting too much and thereby increasing our cancer risk. This is not well studied in the literature, and it is controversial.

Some researchers state that getting a few minutes of sun per day, even to the point of creating "minimal erythema" – a bit of redness to the skin – is beneficial and will not significantly increase skin cancer risk.

This turns out to be about 20 minutes of midday sun for light skinned individuals, and several times that much for people with darker skin. Other researchers state that sun exposure should be absolutely minimized, and suggest that getting vitamin D through the diet should be sufficient.

But even if did want to get all our vitamin D from the sun, it's just not possible for people living in the northern latitudes. Researchers have found that the sun intensity in wintertime is too low for vitamin D synthesis in places like Edmonton, Canada, or Bergen, Norway, or Boston, USA.

For those interested in trying to use sun exposure to ensure adequate vitamin D status while minimizing skin cancer risk, Dr. Michael Holick, writing in his book *The UV Advantage*, offers a comprehensive system. Using tables in the book, one can determine how much sun exposure is necessary at various times of the year for a specific skin type at a specific latitude.

Tanning beds also can allow the body to manufacture vitamin D through the skin. In fact, this might be one reason the tanning industry does so well: apart from increasing pigmentation, tanning treats the vitamin D deficiency that is common in sun-deprived areas in the wintertime, and so makes people feel better. Tanning beds, though, also might increase skin cancer risk overall. Again, there is insufficient evidence to make an absolute statement on this point.

Getting vitamin D in food is not a realistic option, unless you drink a few gallons of milk per day or are willing to eat a few pounds of mushrooms with your breakfast cereal.

What I would suggest, after reviewing the literature and weighing the pros and cons, is that anyone who wants to make sure they get enough vitamin D should take a supplement rather than using sun exposure or tanning beds. Given the uncertainty, it is best to take the safe path.

People have a reluctance to believe that they need to take a nutritional supplement to be healthy. It's not natural, they think.

Well, it's not really natural for tropical apes to be living indoors. It's not natural for African animals to live in Canada without some kind of adaptation to the environment. It's also not natural, by the way, to have a heated house, to eat food grown a few thousand miles from where you live, or to drink bottled water.

And anyway, vitamin D isn't a vitamin. It's a steroid hormone, like estrogen and cortisol, and taking a pill isn't replacing something you should be getting from your diet, it's replacing the sun.

I have found no evidence that taking 2,000 units of storage-form vitamin D per day should have any negative effects for any individual. This dose is approximately what the body needs in a given day. It is below the level of toxicity that even the most paranoid, circumspect analysis of the literature can identify. It is far below levels accidentally given to thousands of dairy customers for a period of years. It is below the 2,400 units per day the National Academy of Sciences, working with sketchy information and with what I believe is an unreasonable level of caution, identifies as the upper safe limit. 2,000 units per day of vitamin D is safe and is enough, in people without an intestinal absorption problem, to bring the body's vitamin D to a healthy level.

This is something that you can do on your own. Vitamin D supplements typically come in 400 unit capsules, and one would have to take five of these per day to reach 2,000 units. However, some manufacturers make 1,000 unit and 2,000 unit capsules, and these are available in some stores. You may have to shop around.

If you want to go the medical route, you can ask your doctor to check a "25-hydroxy vitamin D level," which measures the blood level of the storage form of vitamin D in your body. Your level may come back with a "normal" range listed next to it. Keep in mind that this range is based on the average levels of 25-OH vitamin D in a reference population. "Normal" does not mean the same as "healthy." It is normal to have vitamin D deficiency these days. A strict cutoff for vitamin D deficiency is 20 nanograms per deciliter, or ng/dL. A more reasonable cutoff, which is being used by some labs today, is 32 ng/dL.

You should also remember that your 25-OH vitamin D level will vary with the season, and with how much time you spend outdoors. If you're just back from a vacation in Costa Rica, your level will probably be higher than at the end of winter after you've been working indoors for six months.

If you have vitamin D deficiency, your doctor may choose to prescribe a high dose vitamin D supplement. Generally this comes in the form of capsules containing 50,000 units of storage-form vitamin D, to be taken once per week only. Don't take these pills every day unless your doctor specifically indicates you should. One pill per week for eight weeks should fill up the tank, so to speak, and replenish your vitamin D stores. If your level is still low after the eight weeks, you can try another eight-week course of therapy. If that second course doesn't work, you might have an absorption problem; that's something that might require a visit to a specialist.

Keep in mind that you can safely take 2,000 units of vitamin D per day without visiting your doctor; at this dose, you'll probably get enough, and it won't require any blood tests for monitoring. However, do not take both prescription vitamin D and over-the-counter vitamin D supplements at the same time.

If you have kidney disease, the issue becomes more complicated. The kidneys are what do most of the transforming of storage vitamin D to active vitamin D. Without this transformation, the vitamin D you ingest is not usable.

Once kidney disease gets bad enough, patients have to take an active form of vitamin D. If you want to know if you need it, ask your doctor to check your parathyroid hormone level. That's a hormone that goes into overdrive to keep calcium levels up when there isn't enough vitamin D. If you have kidney disease and parathyroid hormone levels are elevated, you might need to take active vitamin D. The risk of taking active vitamin D is that calcium levels might go too high, and this is relatively easy if you are taking the active form of this hormone.

## 9.1 Children

It is difficult to make recommendations on children's health, because there is so much to gain and so much to lose. One small intervention that can help a child during a crucial time in development can change a life; one small mistake can be catastrophic.

Bringing this thought to bear on vitamin D, it is clear that at least small mistakes are being made in children's nutrition. Rickets, the bone-deforming disease that first appeared in the $17^{th}$ century, is returning, and children arrive at emergency departments with seizures due to low calcium. Among infants, those fed exclusively on breast milk are at highest risk because they get all their nutrition from mothers who may themselves be vitamin D deficient.

On the other hand, reports in the medical literature show that giving children high dose vitamin D supplements can cause a toxic reaction; this too would be a mistake.

We are left with what is probably the safest path, through the middle. Pediatricians now recommend that mothers who are exclusively breastfeeding give their infants 200 units of vitamin D per day. The recommended intake of vitamin D for children is 400 units, and the tolerable upper intake, according to the National Academies of Science, is 1000 units. As for adults, the true level inducing toxicity is probably higher, but we should hold to what is known to be safe.

*"Knowledge is a light that God projects into the heart of the Knower."*
- Ibn al-ʿArabi

# 10. Ethical considerations

## 10.1 Race

Any human being with dark pigment will be at a disadvantage in areas with little sun exposure if vitamin D is not replaced. Without vitamin D or sunlight, these individuals and their children will tend to develop mental illnesses, autoimmune diseases, and will have heart disease and cancer at a higher risk than lighter-pigmented individuals. These statements arise directly out of the evidence presented in chapter 4. People with these illnesses will not do as well in the economy, and may therefore be poorer. In turn, the effects of vitamin D deficiency may be interpreted by individuals in power in terms of race, rather than in terms of biology. In other words, vitamin D deficiency may contribute to racism.

Correcting vitamin D deficiency in individuals with darker pigment – currently in America, this tends to mean "minorities" – therefore can help contribute to equality of opportunity, and perhaps harmony between the races.

An obstacle to addressing this public health problem in the United States is widespread mistrust with which African-American people tend to view the medical establishment. This leads to them not listening to public health messages. Medicine is part of the system that is perceived to keep them down, to oppress them, to deny them opportunity. This attitude is partially related to the Tuskegee Syphilis study, something that many white Americans know little or nothing about. In the Tuskegee study, which ran from 1932 to 1972 in Alabama, researchers with the United States Public Health Service observed the long-term effects of untreated syphilis in 399 African-American males. Researchers told the participants they were being treated for "bad blood," while in fact they were receiving no treatment whatsoever.

Convincing African-Americans to trust a public health message, given the history of this study, is at best difficult. No message presented as "fact" can be accepted without acknowledging the formidable emotional barriers that now exist.

## 10.2 Poverty

Vitamin D deficiency is both a cause and an effect of poverty. The diseases it brings remove individuals from the economy, or decrease their ability to participate in any prosperity. These diseases cost money to treat, and in the United States particularly health care is not universally available. Illness brings poverty, and in poverty one cannot cure illness.

The absence of sunlight therefore is a drain on economies, bringing down the standard of living of nations. It is wrapped up in the complex of poverty, spreading its roots into all facets of physical, emotional and spiritual life. By treating the absence of sunlight, by treating vitamin D deficiency in anyone, we therefore bring all of us to a better place.

## 10.3 Unnecessary suffering

"Pain is a more terrible lord of mankind than even death itself,"said physician Albert Schweitzer. People in severe pain want to die, and death is a release to them. If pain is an evil, then unnecessary pain is a greater one.

The magnitude of unnecessary pain brought about by vitamin D deficiency is unfathomable. Who can count the number of elderly in nursing homes who can't walk solely because of this disease? How can one measure the sum of their emotional pain of immobility and social separation? Add together all the individuals who have aching, body-wide pain due to lack of sunlight. Count the tears of all the relatives of people who have died because vitamin D deficiency was the one additional factor that tipped them into fatal cancer. How many people spend their lives in psychiatric hospitals that might have been just well enough not to be institutionalized had their mothers not been vitamin D deficiency during pregnancy?

*"The world's darkening never reaches to the light of Being."*
  – Martin Heidegger

# 11. Vitamin D in human history

It is difficult to do more than hypothesize about vitamin D as a factor in human history. This area has not been studied, and may be impossible to study directly. However I'd like to offer a few thoughts.

First, it is clear that the varieties of human skin pigmentation exist at least partly due to the need for vitamin D. Most dramatically, in areas of low sunlight, pale skin has evolved in order to reduce the sickness and early death that come from vitamin D deficiency.

Second, human migration patterns reflect a subconscious desire for a normalized vitamin D status. Currently in the United States, for example, a large scale population shift is occurring toward the southern and western states – subtropical and arid areas where sun exposure is more intense and where, therefore, people feel a greater sense of well-being. The reaction toward the profound effects of reversing this metabolic deficiency can manifest itself as contempt for the "bad weather" up north, a cultural separation in which everything from the most mundane elements of daily life to the most rarified political concepts are seen with different eyes.

Areas with Mediterranean and tropical climates have always been desirable places to live, and have been subject to frequent invasions and population displacements: Italy is an example, experiencing waves of migration over the centuries.

Long-term survival of humans in arctic and sub-arctic regions has been possible only when inhabitants find a supplemental source of vitamin D, such as through eating fish or the fat of marine mammals. These food sources are traditional simply because they correct what would otherwise be a life-altering, and frequently life-ending metabolic problem. When dietary patterns change to a more "Western" approach, it should be expected that health should suffer, as seen currently in Eskimo populations.

The domination of the Vikings in northern Europe during the Middle Ages may have been facilitated by dietary practices: the consumption of relatively large amounts of fish may have provided a strength and vigor that provided an advantage versus other European populations.

Industrialization in Europe may have received a boost once cod liver oil use became common to prevent rickets; this would have added mental clarity and energy to the work force, and reduced the economically disadvantageous effects of chronic disease.

*"Imagine you're a space alien looking down on Earth. You have these humans who evolved in the Horn of Africa, as nudists living around the equator. They would have been getting lots of vitamin D through their skin. Then they suddenly … move north and put on lots of clothes and block out most of their capacity to make vitamin D. For me, it's a no-brainer. We're not getting enough."*
- Dr. Reinhold Vieth

# 12. Conclusion

The epidemic of vitamin D deficiency creates a burden of suffering that falls below the radar screen of modern medicine and, for the most part, public health. Economic factors lead the medical community to focus on treatments that can generate revenue, and targeted at people who can pay money. Vitamin D in its natural form is not patentable, and so companies cannot recoup investments in research, development and marketing. Furthermore, an ongoing scientific bias away from discovering and using nutritional remedies for diseases works against this problem being addressed. So the mass of suffering related to this epidemic is unlikely to be aggressively addressed by standard medical and public health practice. It is almost a cultural shift that is necessary: the development of a person-to-person tradition, based on science, allowing the human species to maximize its health by normalizing this metabolic system.

The pathology of vitamin D deficiency disproportionately falls upon minority communities in the developed world: dark-skinned natives, citizens and immigrants who arrive in America and Europe from other countries.

The evidence for this epidemic is somewhat circumstantial, but nonetheless quite strong. The cure for this epidemic is extremely low risk – 2,000 units per day of vitamin D in oral form.

Public health officials are naturally careful about making sweeping generalizations due to the possibility of doing harm to a vast number of people. However, from a clinical perspective, it is clear to me that for the average individual, supplementation of 2,000 units per day is safe and very likely to offer profound benefits to health.

# NOTES

[1] Jablonski NG and Chaplin G. The evolution of human skin coloration. J. Hum. Evol. 39:57-106, 2000.

[2] Mayow J. Rachitidologia, or a tract of the disease rhachitis, commonly called rickets. Oxford, 1685.

[3] Rajakumar K. Vitamin D, cod-liver oil, sunlight, and rickets: a historical perspective. Pediatrics 112:e132-3135, 2003.

[4] Dunn PM. Francis Glisson (1597-1677) and the "discovery" of rickets. Archives of Disease in Childhood 78(2):154F-155F, 1998.

[5] Dunn PM. Professor Armand Trousseau (1801-67) and the treatment of rickets. Archives of Disease in Childhood 80(2):155F-157F, 1999.

[6] Hardy A. Commentary: bread and alum, syphilis and sunlight: rickets in the nineteenth century. International Journal of Epidemiology 32:340-341, 2003.

[7] Kaper BP, Romness MJ and Urbanek PJ. Nutritional rickets: report of four cases diagnosed at orthopedic evaluation. American Journal of Orthopedics 29(3):214-218, 2000.

[8] Malabanan A, Veronikis IE and Holick MF. Redefining Vitamin D deficiency. Lancet 351(9105):805-6, 1998.

[9] Thomas, MK, Lloyd-Jones DM, Thadhani RI et al. Hypovitaminosis D in medical inpatients. New England Journal of Medicine 338(12):777-783, 1998.

[10] Chapuy MC, Preziosi P, Maamer M et al. Prevalence of vitamin D insufficiency in an adult normal population. Osteoporosis International 7:439-443, 1997.

[11] Isaia G, Giorgino R, Rini GB et al. Prevalence of hypovitaminosis D in elderly women in Italy: clinical consequences and risk factors. Osteoporosis International 14:577-582, 2003.

[12] Harris SS, Soteriades E, Coolidge JAS et al. Vitamin D insufficiency and hyperparathyroidism in a low income, multiracial, elderly population. Journal of Clinical Endocrinology and Metabolism 85:4125-4130, 2000.

[13] Du X, Greenfield H, Fraser DR et al. Vitamin D deficiency and associated factors in adolescent girls in Beijing. American Journal of Clinical Nutrition 74(4):4940500, 2001.

[14] Bassir M, Laborie S, Lapillonne A et al. Vitamin D deficiency in Iranian mothers and their neonates: a pilot study. Acta Paediatrica 90(5):577-9, 2001.

[15] Wielders JPM, van Dormael PD, Eskes PF and Duk, M J. Severe vitamin-D deficiency in more than half of the immigrant pregnant women of non-western origin and their newborns. Nederlands Tijdschrift voor Geneeskunde 150(9):495-9, 2006.

[16] Garland FC, Garland CF, Gorham ED and Young JF. Geographic variation in breast cancer mortality in the United States: a hypothesis involving exposure to solar radiation. Preventive Medicine 19:614-622, 1990.

[17] Emerson JC and Weiss NS. Colorectal cancer and solar radiation. Cancer Causes and Control 3:95-99, 1992.

[18] Hanchette CL and Schwartz GG. Geographic patterns of prostate cancer mortality. Cancer 70:2861-2869, 1992.

[19]     LaPorte RE, Tajima N, Akerblom HK et al. Geographic differences in the risk of insulin-dependent diabetes mellitus: the importance of registries. Diabetes Care 8 (suppl. 1):101-107, 1985.

[20]     Freedman DM, Dosemeci M and Alavanja MCR. Mortality from multiple sclerosis and exposure to residential and occupational solar radiation: a case-control study based on death certificates. Occupational and Environmental Medicine 57:418-421, 2000.

[21]     Templer DI, Regier MW and Corgiat MD. Similar distribution of schizophrenia and multiple sclerosis. Journal of Clinical Psychiatry 46(2):73, 1985.

[22]     Gloth FM 3rd, Alam W and Hollis B. Vitamin D vs broad spectrum phototherapy in the treatment of seasonal affective disorder. Journal of Nutrition, Health & Aging. 3(1):5-7, 1999.

[23]     Lansdowne AT and Provost SC. Vitamin D3 enhances mood in healthy subjects during winter. Psychopharmacology. 135(4):319-23, 1998.

[24]     Mackay-Sim A, Feron F, Eyles D and McGrath BT. Schizophrenia, vitamin D, and brain development. International Review of Neurobiology. 59:351-80, 2004.

[25]     Stene LC and Joner G. Norwegian Childhood Diabetes Study Group. Use of cod liver oil during the first year of life is associated with lower risk of childhood-onset type 1 diabetes: a large, population-based, case-control study. American Journal of Clinical Nutrition. 78(6):1128-34, 2003.

[26]     Giarratana N, Penna G, Amuchastegui S, et al. A vitamin D analog down-regulates proinflammatory chemokine production by pancreatic islets inhibiting T cell recruitment and type 1 diabetes development. Journal of Immunology. 173(4):2280-7, 2004.

[27]     Merlino LA, Curtis J, Mikuls TR et al. Iowa Women's Health Study. Vitamin D intake is inversely associated with rheumatoid arthritis: results from the Iowa Women's Health Study. Arthritis & Rheumatism. 50(1):72-7, 2004.

[28]     Andjelkovic Z, Vojinovic J, Pejnovic N et al. Disease modifying and immunomodulatory effects of high dose 1 alpha (OH) D3 in rheumatoid arthritis patients. Clinical & Experimental Rheumatology. 17(4):453-6, 1999.

[29]     Kamen DL, Cooper GS, Bouali H et al. Vitamin D deficiency in systemic lupus erythematosus. Autoimmunity Reviews. 5(2):114-7, 2006.

[30]     Munger KL, Zhang SM, O'Reilly E, et al. Vitamin D Intake and Incidence of Multiple Sclerosis. Neurology 62:60-65,2004.

[31]     John EM, Schwartz GG, Dreon DM and Koo J. Vitamin D and breast cancer risk: the NHANES I Epidemiologic follow-up study, 1971-1975 to 1992. National Health and Nutrition Examination Survey. Cancer Epidemiology, Biomarkers & Prevention. 8(5):399-406, 1999.

[32]     Beer TM, Eilers KM, Garzotto M et al. Weekly High-Dose Calcitriol and Docetaxel in Metastatic Androgen-Independent Prostate Cancer. Journal of Clinical Oncology 21(1):123-128, 2003.

[33]     Prabhala A, Garg R and Dandona P. Severe myopathy associated with vitamin D deficiency in western New York. Archives of Internal Medicine. 160(8):1199-203, 2000.

[34]     Flicker L, MacInnis RJ, Stein MS et al. Should older people in residential care receive vitamin D to prevent falls? Results of a randomized trial. Journal of the American Geriatrics Society. 53(11):1881-8, 2005.

[35]     Plotnikoff GA and Quigley JM. Prevalence of severe hypovitaminosis D in patients with persistent, nonspecific musculoskeletal pain. Mayo Clinic Proceedings. 78(12):1463-70, 2003.

36       Holick MF. Vitamin D deficiency: what a pain it is. Mayo Clinic Proceedings. 78(12):1457-9, 2003.

37       Al Faraj S and Al Mutairi K. Vitamin D deficiency and chronic low back pain in Saudi Arabia. Spine. 28(2):177-9, 2003 Jan.

38       Li YC, Qiao G, Uskokovic M et al. Vitamin D: a negative endocrine regulator of the renin-angiotensin system and blood pressure. Journal of Steroid Biochemistry & Molecular Biology. 89-90(1-5):387-92, 2004.

39       Kamycheva E, Joakimsen RM and Jorde R. Intakes of calcium and vitamin D predict body mass index in the population of northern Norway. Journal of Nutrition 132:102-106, 2002.

40       Arunabh S, Pollack S, Yeh J and Aloia JF. Body fat content and 25-hydroxyvitamin D levels in healthy women. Journal of Clinical Endocrinology and Metabolism 88: 157-161, 2003.

# Index

Africa .................. 9, 10, 12, 37, 40, 44, 51, 54, 56, 57, 61, 62, 67, 68, 72

angiotensin ................................................................................................. 43

arthritis ........................................................... 6, 19, 20, 36, 37, 52

beriberi ................................................................................................ 15

bone .................. 6, 9, 13-15, 19, 20, 21, 33, 36, 39, 42, 44, 51, 64

brain ............................................ 9, 10, 15, 18, 21, 33, 34, 37, 72

calcipotriene .......................................................................... 25

calcium ........................ 13, 14, 17, 20, 21, 25, 37, 42, 54, 64, 65

cancer .................. 6, 10, 11, 28-31, 35, 38, 39, 43, 54, 55, 56, 61, 62, 67, 68

cholecalciferol .................................................................................. 7

cod liver oil ................................................ 15, 16, 23, 36, 71

cohort studies .......................................................... 27, 28, 38

darkness ..................................................... 47, 48, 49, 53

depression .......................................... 1, 20, 33, 34, 48, 52

diabetes ...................................................... 6, 32, 36, 40, 56

economics ................................................................... 9, 24

ergocalciferol ............................................ 7, 25, 39, 40, 52

evolution ........................................ 9, 10, 11, 12, 13, 18, 61

fish ...................................................... 12, 16, 23, 49, 70, 71

folic acid ........................................................................ 11

food ...................... ix, 12, 13, 16, 17, 18, 23, 37, 48, 51, 55, 56, 62, 63, 70

hair ........................................................... 2, 10, 40, 55

heart ...................................... 18, 21, 29, 36, 43, 49, 67

height ........................................................................ 6, 44

hormone .................. 2, 5, 7, 13, 18, 19, 20, 21, 23, 33, 36, 43, 47, 63, 64

iguanas ........................................................................ 13

immune system ......................................... 9, 18, 21, 35

light .......... 2, 5-7, 9-15, 18, 22, 31-34, 36-43, 47-49, 53, 56, 57, 61, 62, 67, 68, 70

lupus ...................................................... 6, 10, 37, 48

melanin ........................................................................ 9, 10 milk.................................................. 7, 17, 23, 53, 59, 60, 61, 62, 65

mood................................................. 2, 21, 30, 33, 34, 49, 56

multiple sclerosis............................... 10, 32, 36, 37, 38, 54

muscle...............................6, 9, 10, 14, 19, 21, 29, 39, 40, 41, 42, 52, 55

mushrooms ........................................................... 23, 24, 62

Native Americans................................................................13

nutrition...................1, 5, 7, 15, 16, 18, 23, 25, 38, 40, 41, 51, 52, 54, 62, 64, 65, 72

obesity................................................................................ 9, 44

osteoporosis........................................ 1, 6, 9, 19, 21, 22, 25, 29, 39, 54

pain....................................... 1, 6, 9, 20, 21, 29, 33, 36, 40, 41, 42, 49, 51, 52, 54, 68

parathyroid hormone........................................................ 21, 64

patent ......................................................... 2, 6, 24, 25, 39, 43, 72

Phenomenology................................................................... 9, 47

phosphate.......................................................................... 21, 42

phototherapy....................................................................... 33, 34

psoriasis ......................................................................... 25, 42, 43

public health................................ 2, 5, 9, 10, 13, 16, 28, 54, 55, 56, 59, 67, 68, 72, 73

randomized controlled trials........................................... 27, 28

RDA ........................................................................ 47, 53, 57, 60

rickets................................. 9, 13, 14, 15, 16, 17, 20, 33, 44, 64, 71

schizophrenia............................................................... 6, 32, 34

scurvy ............................................................................... 15, 23

seasonal affective disorder............................................... 9, 33

skin .......2, 5, 6, 7, 9-12, 14, 18, 20, 23, 25, 41-43, 49, 52, 53, 55, 56, 61, 62, 70, 72

steroid ..............................................2, 5, 7, 9, 18, 19, 20, 33, 47, 56, 63

strength.............................. 6, 7, 27, 38, 39, 40, 44, 48, 49, 52, 55, 71

sunlight .............. 2, 6, 9, 11-15, 18, 22, 31-33, 36, 37, 39, 43, 53, 56, 57, 61, 67-70

terminology........................................................................6, 9

toxicity ........................................... 29, 54, 56, 59, 60, 63, 65

Tuskegee Syphilis study......................................................67

ultraviolet..............................................7, 9-11, 12, 13, 31, 43, 61

# The author

Michael D. Merrill attended Dartmouth College as an undergraduate, and worked as a journalist in the 1980's, receiving a master's degree in journalism from Columbia University in 1987. He attended medical school and residency, and received a master's degree in epidemiology at the State University of New York (SUNY) at Buffalo. He is clinical instructor in the departments of Medicine and Preventive Medicine at the School of Medicine and in the School of Pharmacy at SUNY–Buffalo. He is board certified in Internal Medicine and Preventive Medicine. He writes a monthly freelance health column for the *Buffalo News*.

Printed in the United States
96105LV00005B/247-249/A

9 781430 305743